Aaruni Saxena

Insight into Aspirin and NSAIDs interactions

Aaruni Saxena

Insight into Aspirin and NSAIDs interactions

Südwestdeutscher Verlag für Hochschulschriften

Impressum / Imprint

Bibliografische Information der Deutschen Nationalbibliothek: Die Deutsche Nationalbibliothek verzeichnet diese Publikation in der Deutschen Nationalbibliografie; detaillierte bibliografische Daten sind im Internet über http://dnb.d-nb.de abrufbar.
Alle in diesem Buch genannten Marken und Produktnamen unterliegen warenzeichen-, marken- oder patentrechtlichem Schutz bzw. sind Warenzeichen oder eingetragene Warenzeichen der jeweiligen Inhaber. Die Wiedergabe von Marken, Produktnamen, Gebrauchsnamen, Handelsnamen, Warenbezeichnungen u.s.w. in diesem Werk berechtigt auch ohne besondere Kennzeichnung nicht zu der Annahme, dass solche Namen im Sinne der Warenzeichen- und Markenschutzgesetzgebung als frei zu betrachten wären und daher von jedermann benutzt werden dürften.

Bibliographic information published by the Deutsche Nationalbibliothek: The Deutsche Nationalbibliothek lists this publication in the Deutsche Nationalbibliografie; detailed bibliographic data are available in the Internet at http://dnb.d-nb.de.
Any brand names and product names mentioned in this book are subject to trademark, brand or patent protection and are trademarks or registered trademarks of their respective holders. The use of brand names, product names, common names, trade names, product descriptions etc. even without a particular marking in this work is in no way to be construed to mean that such names may be regarded as unrestricted in respect of trademark and brand protection legislation and could thus be used by anyone.

Coverbild / Cover image: www.ingimage.com

Verlag / Publisher:
Südwestdeutscher Verlag für Hochschulschriften
ist ein Imprint der / is a trademark of
OmniScriptum GmbH & Co. KG
Bahnhofstraße 28, 66111 Saarbrücken, Deutschland / Germany
Email: info@svh-verlag.de

Herstellung: siehe letzte Seite /
Printed at: see last page
ISBN: 978-3-8381-5025-3

Zugl. / Approved by: Müster:Düsseldorf, Universität Düsseldorf,2014

Copyright © 2014 OmniScriptum GmbH & Co. KG
Alle Rechte vorbehalten. / All rights reserved. Saarbrücken 2014

Publications in relation to the thesis:

1. Hohlfeld T, Saxena A, Schrör K. High on treatment platelet reactivity against aspirin by non-steroidal anti-inflammatory drugs - pharmacological mechanisms and clinical relevance. Thromb Haemost, 2013,109:825-33

Abstracts (peer reviewed):

1. Hohlfeld T, Saxena A, Schrör K (2010) Drug-drug interactions at the level of platelet cyclooxygenase. Med Chem Res 19: S20. (Presented at CTDDR Current Trends in Drug Discovery Research Feb. 26-28, 2010 in Lucknow, India)

2. Hohlfeld T, Pott A, Saxena A, Ledwoch C, Rauch B H, Schrör K (2011) Interaction of Free Fatty Acids with Platelet Inhibition by Aspirin. Arteriosc Thromb Vasc Biol, ATVB Conference Abstracs Supplement, P663. (Presented at ATVB Conference, Chicago, US, April 30, 2011)

3. Saxena A, Weber H, Schrör K, Hohlfeld T (2011) Remarkable Differences in the Effect of Individual Nonsteroidal Anti-Inflammatory Drugs on the Antiplatelet Action of Aspirin. Circulation 124 (Suppl. S): A10243. (Presented on 71st AHA scientific sessions Orlando,Fluorida, USA, Nov 13-15, 2011)

4. Saxena A, Kurt M, Schrör K, Hohlfeld T (2012) Insight from molecular modeling into the drug/drug interaction of nonsteriodal anti-inflammatory drugs with the antiplatelet effect of aspirin. Clin Res Cardiol 101 (Suppl 1): P1720. (Presented at 78th Annual Meeting of the German Cardiac Society, Mannheim, Germany on April 11-14, 2012)

5. Saxena A, Gohlke H, Singh S, Schrör K, Hohlfeld T (2012) Drug-Drug Interactions Between Aspirin and NSAIDs are Predicted by Kinetics of Cyclooxygenase-1 Inhibition. Circulation 126:A9050. (Presented at AHA 72nd Scientific sessions, Los Angeles, US, Nov 2-7, 2012)

Papers under review:

1. Saxena A, Balaramnavar MV, Hohlfeld T, Saxena AK. Drug/Drug interaction of common NSAIDs with antiplatelet effect of aspirin in human platelets. Eur J Pharmacol.

Further scientific publications:

1. Saxena A, Tyagi K, Muller SC, Drewelow B.Quantitative pharmacokinetic patients relationship (QPPR) for piperacillin-tazobactam during continuous venovenous heamodialysis/filtration. Med Chem Res, 2008, 17: 199 – 204

SUMMARY

This thesis studies the interaction of aspirin (acetylsalicylic acid, ASA) and nonsteroidal antiinflammatory drugs (NSAIDs) in human blood platelets. ASA is widely used all around the globe to prevent atherothrombotic events. Multi-morbid patients suffering from cardiovascular and rheumatological disorders including rheumatoid arthritis or osteoarthritis need a comedication of ASA with NSAID drugs. Hence, potential NSAID/ASA drug interactions, possibly affecting the cardioprotective effect of ASA, are of great interest. The present research aimed to determine which NSAIDs would decrease the anti-platelet activity of ASA.

Using arachidonic acid-induced platelet aggregation and thromboxane formation[108] in platelet rich plasma from healthy donors, the effect of NSAIDs on the antiplatelet activity of ASA was studied experimentally. It turned out that celecoxib, dipyrone, fenoprofen, flufenamic acid, ibuprofen, methylaminoantipyrin, mefenamic acid, nabumetone, naproxen, nimesulide, NS-398, oxaprozin, phenazone, piroxicam, propylphenazone, sulindac sulfide and tolmetin clearly decreased the antiplatelet activity of ASA. In contrast, acetaminophen, diclofenac, flurbiprofen, indomethacin and ketoprofen did not decrease the antiplatelet activity of ASA. The data was further used to design a QSAR model which showed that the IC_{50} and selectivity of NSAID towards COX-1 might predict the effect of NSAID on the antiplatelet activity of ASA.

Further investigation aimed to identify the reasons for the interference of NSAIDs with the antiplatelet activity of ASA by molecular docking studies, which were performed for all NSAIDs on COX-I protein (PDB ID: 1CQE). Docking studies suggested that NSAIDs, forming hydrogen bonds with Ser 530, Arg 120, Tyr 385 and some other amino acids in the COX-I hydrophobic channel, play role in determining whether a particular NSAID might decrease the antiplatelet activity of ASA or not. NSAIDs which decreased the antiplatelet activity of ASA in the in vitro experiments mostly showed one or more hydrogen bond interactions with Ser 530, Tyr 385 or Arg 120. Less or no hydrogen bond interactions were seen in docking studies of NSAIDs which did not decrease the antiplatelet activity of ASA in the in vitro experiments.

Therefore, hydrogen bond interactions with Ser 530 and Tyr 385 were found to be most relevant for NSAIDs effects on the antiplatelet activity of ASA.

ABBREVIATIONS

ASA	Aspirin
CAMD	Computer assisted molecular design
COX	Cyclooxygenase
COX-I	Cyclooxygenase 1
COX-II	Cyclooxygenase 2
DE	Differential Evolution
DF	Degree of freedom
ED_{50}	Effective dose showing effect in 50% population
GFA	Genetic function approximation
G/PLS	Genetic partial least squares
HHU	Henrich- Heine- University in Duesseldorf
IC_{50}	Inhibitory concentration for half maximal
ICM	Internal Coordinates Mechanics
IR	Infrared
LFER	Linear free energy relationship
MAA	Methyl amino antipyrin
MC	Monte carlo
MD	Molecular dynamic
MR	Molar refractivity
MLR	Multiple linear regression
MV	Molar volume
MVD	Molegro virtual docker
MW	Molecular weight
NF-kB	Nuclear factor kappa-light-chain-enhancer of activated B cells
NMR	Nuclear magnetic resonance
NSAID	Non-steriodal anti-inflammatory drugs
PCA	Principal component analysis
PDB	Protein data bank
PGE_2	Prostglandin E2 ((5Z,11α,13E,15S)-7-[3-hydroxy-2-(3-hydroxyoct-1-enyl)- 5-oxo-cyclopentyl] hept-5-enoic acid)
PGI_2	Prostacyclin I2 ((Z)-5-[(4R,5R)-5-hydroxy-4-((S,E)-3-hydroxyoct-1-enyl)hexahydro-2H-cyclopenta[b]furan-2-ylidene]pentanoic acid)
PLP	Piecewise linear potential
PLS	Partial least square
PRP	Platelet rich plasma
QSAR	Quantitative structural analysis and relationship
SD	Standard deviation
TXB_2	Thromboxane
Vr	Van der Waal's radius
Vw	Van der Waal's volum

INDEX

Abbreviations	**V**
1 Introduction	**2**
1.1 Historical summary of aspirin	2
1.2 General mechanism of action of aspirin and other NSAIDs	4
1.3 Molecular mechanism of aspirin action	4
1.4 Antiplatelet action of aspirin and non-aspirin NSAIDs	6
1.5 Drug/drug interactions between NSAIDs and aspirin	7
1.6 Computer aided molecular docking, molecular design and QSAR	8
1.7 Aims of the study	10
2 Materials and Methods	**11**
2.1 Drugs & chemicals	11
2.2 Platelet aggregation and thromboxane formation	12
2.3 Molecular modeling and in silico docking	13
2.4 Mathematical model (QSAR)	14
2.5 Statistical evaluation of the experimental results	18
3 Results	**19**
3.1 Experimental results	19
3.2 QSAR results	27
3.3 Docking results	31
4 Discussion	**46**
4.1 Discussion of experimental results	47
4.2 QSAR results discussion	50
4.3 Docking results discussion	50
4.4 Discussion of clinical implications	54
4.5 Criticism of Methodology	55
5 Conclusion	**57**
6 References	**58**
7 Curriculum Vitae	**68**
8 Acknowledgments	**69**

1. INTRODUCTION

Medicine has evolved drastically impressively during the last years and numerous new drugs which more specifically target particular diseases have become milestones in medical progress. One particular drug, commonly regarded as an ´old´ one, is acetylsalicylic acid (ASA), also named aspirin. ASA has obtained a broad area for application and use. It is effective, relatively safe, inexpensive and one of the most intensively studied and most frequently used drugs worldwide for prevention of cardiovascular diseases[1].

Starting more than 100 years ago as an analgesic and antipyretic, ASA has proved to be effective in the prevention of myocardial infarction, stroke and peripheral vascular disease. Beyond atherothrombotic disorders, ASA appears also effective in the prevention of different types of diseases including cancer especially colorectal carcinoma[2].

The way ASA has proved effective in so many diseases makes a fascinating story. Besides ASA, non-steroidal anti-inflammatory drugs (NSAIDs) including ibuprofen, diclofenac and many others have been developed to specifically target inflammatory diseases, pain and fever. NSAIDs also are among the most common used drugs, some of which available free of prescription in many countries.

Administration of more medicines to multi-morbid patients exponentially increases the number of potential drug/drug interactions. These are a common cause of unwanted drug effects[3]. Specifically, numerous earlier reports suggested that NSAIDs may prevent the antiplatelet action of ASA and thereby cause "aspirin resistance" or "high on-treatment platelet reactivity". Health agencies (e.g., Food and Drug Administration) released warnings in this context[4]. The interaction between ASA and a number of NSAID drugs is the subject of this thesis.

1.1 Historical summary of aspirin

ASA has been manufactured and marketed since 1899. Several other medicinal products have been used for treatment of pain and fever, some derived from willow and salicylate rich plants. An Ancient Egyptian text shows reference to willow and myrth (a salicylate plant) with analgesic and antipyretic properties[5]. Willow bark preparations were used already by Hippocrates in 5th century BC for reducing fever and pain in children.

Edward Stone (1702–1768) described the potential of willow bark extract to cure the symptoms including fatigue, fever and pain especially in patients suffering with malaria[5].

Advancements in organic chemistry in the 19th century enabled to isolate salicin, the β-glycoside of salicylic acid. Joseph Buchner (1813-1879) obtained salicin crystals in 1828. The Italian scientists Brugnatelli and Fontana considered salicin as the active component of willow bark. During the 19th century, interest grew to learn more about salicin, salicylic acid, and sodium salicylate. The French scientist Leroux obtained in 1830 for the first time salicin in crystalline form [5].

Further steps in research on ASA were taken in Elberfeld, Germany, at the Bayer company. A new research group which included the scientists Heinrich Dreser, Arthur Eichengrün and Felix Hoffman took the project for development of acetylsalicylic acid as drug ASA in order to improve efficacy and tolerability of salicylic acid[5,6]. Finally in 1897, Hoffman advised a better method of forming ASA from salicyclic acid refluxed with acetic anhydride[5]. Bayer company mentioned in 1897 that the active ingredient in ASA, acetylsalicylic acid, was synthesized for the first time in a chemically pure and thus stable form[5,7].

The prevention of myocardial infarction and stroke is attributed to early work by Paul Gibson and Lawrence Craven[8]. Gibson recognised in 1948 that ASA reduces the ability of platelets to aggregate[9]. Ten years later, Craven demonstrated by an observational study that this effect may be exploited to prevent heart attacks and myocardial infarction[10]. Later landmark trials (e.g., ISIS-2 study, Physician's health study) substantially supported the usefulness of ASA for secondary prevention of myocardial infarction and stroke[11,12]. The mechanism of action of ASA has been elucidated by John Vane, who (together with Bergström and Samuelsson) earned the Nobel prize in 1982[13].

ASA derives its name from a chemical name of acetylsalicylic acid, also known as Acetylspirsäure in German. Spirsäure (salicylic acid) was named for a particular type of plant species known as Spirea ulmaria. From this plant ASA could be successfully derived [14].

1.2 General mechanism of action of aspirin and other NSAIDs

ASA and other NSAIDs inhibit prostaglandin synthesis by inhibiting cyclooxygenase (COX) enzymes, resulting in many physiological and pathological effects[15]. The analgesic, antipyretic and antiphlogistic effects of ASA and other NSAIDs are particularly well characterized. Prostaglandins (PGE2, PGI2) are known to increase pain receptor sensitivity and thereby cause hyperalgesia. NSAIDs decrease prostaglandin synthesis and prevent prostaglandin induced hyperalgesia[15]. Another effect of prostaglandins involves central temperature regulation, resulting in fever. By inhibition of prostaglandin synthesis, NSAIDs are anti-pyretic agents. Some prostaglandins play an important role as inflammation mediators in addition to histamine and bradykinin. NSAIDs help to control inflammation by inhibiting prostaglandin synthesis. Moreover, several prostaglandins modulate vascular tone either by vasodilation (PGI_2, PGE_2) or vasoconstriction (TXA_2, PGE_2, $PGF_{2\alpha}$). Many other effects of prostaglandins are known. Their discussion would exceed the scope of this introduction.

1.3 Molecular mechanism of aspirin action

Therapeutic effects of ASA include reduction of inflammation, analgesia, antipyresis as well as prevention of arterial thrombosis. These are mainly (but not exclusively) attributed to the fact that ASA decreases the production of prostaglandins and thromboxane. ASA irreversibly inactivates the cyclooxygenase (COX) enzyme, which is the common initial step of synthesis of prostaglandin and thromboxane[16].

There are two types of cyclooxygenase, cyclooxygenase-1 (COX-1) and cyclooxygenase-2 (COX-2). Recent research has also suggested the potential existence of additional subspecies of COX-enzymes, such as COX-2a and others[17]. ASA inhibits both COX-1 and COX-2, while it is more potent on COX-1[18]. All COX isoforms are involved in generation of prostaglandins and thromboxane. Prostaglandins are considered as pro-inflammatory and increasing sensitivity for pain.

ASA irreversibly inhibits COX enzymes[16,19] by acetylation of a serine residue (Ser 530) within the hydrophobic substrate channel of COX, near the active site[20]. The molecular mechanism of COX acetylation by ASA is shown in figure 1.

Figure 1. Initial complex formation of aspirin with the amino acids Tyr 385, Ser 530 and Arg120 at the substrate channel of COX-1. This is an essential step of the molecular action of aspirin, which ultimately leds to COX acetylation and inhibition.

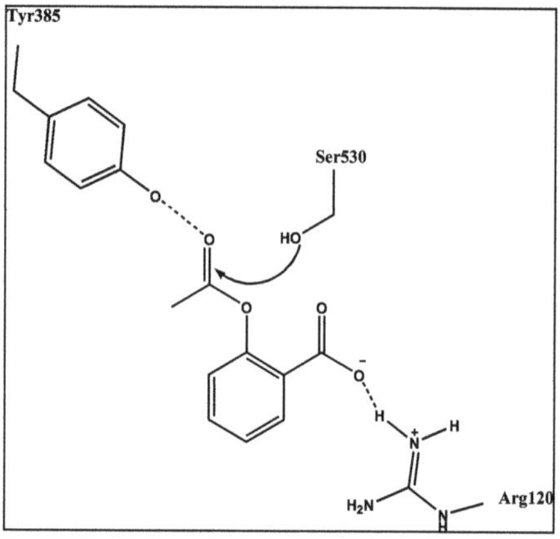

Irreversible inhibition of COX is peculiar to ASA and it makes ASA different from other NSAIDs, such as diclofenac and ibuprofen, which are reversible inhibitors[21].

As a consequence, acetylation of the COX enzyme prevents the access of arachidonic acid to the catalytic site within the substrate channel of COX enzyme, resulting in inhibition of the synthesis of PGG_2 and PGH_2, as well as formation of subsequent prostaglandins (PGI_2, PG_E, $PGF_{2\alpha}$ and PGD_2) and thromboxane in different cells and tissues.

Apart from COX inhibition, ASA shows additional modes of action. For example, ASA uncouples mitochondrial oxidative phosphorylation, induces nitric oxid formation, inhibits coagulation and reduces leukocyte adhesion. Recent research has also shown that salicyclic acid formed by ASA deacetylation modulates signaling through NF-kB (nuclear factor kappa-light-chain-enhancer of activated B cells)[22].

ASA may cause numerous side effects, including bleeding, gastric ulcers[23], ASA induced asthma[24] and Reye syndrome[25]. These are likely dependent on the dose, which explains that different doses of ASA are associated with specific effects (table 1).

Table 1: Dose-dependent effects of ASA (modified from reference 26)

Effects of ASA	ASA dose required
Inhibition of Platelet aggregation	73-300 mg/day
Analgesic/ antipyretic	1 g single or multiple doses
Antiphlogistic	6-8 g/ day

1.4 Anti-platelet action of aspirin and non-aspirin NSAIDs

Thromboxane is required for platelet thrombus formation. Decreased synthesis of thromboxane reduces the risk of resulting thrombose formation and myocardial infraction[27,28]. Prostacyclin is a functional antagonist since it potently inhibits platelet function. Both prostaglandins also exert opposite effects on vascular tone (Table 2). Hence, the inhibition of thromboxane formation (ideally without altering prostacyclin synthesis) is the concept for the use of aspirin in secondary prevention of atherothrombotic events.

Table 2: Basic characteristics of thromboxane and prostacyclin in the vascular system.

Eicosanoid	Thromboxane	Prostacyclin
site of formation	mainly platelets macrophages other vascular cells	endothelium smooth muscle
COX isoform	COX-1	COX-1 and COX-2
Biological function	increase in platelet aggregation, vasoconstriction	increase in platelet aggregation, vasodilation

Even at a low dose of 70–100 mg/day, ASA irreversibly blocks platelet COX-1 as described above, resulting in decreased thromboxane synthesis[29]. Platelets are particularly sensitive to inhibition by aspirin because of several reasons. First, anucleate platelets do not have a relevant protein synthesis. This means that once a platelet has acetylated COX-1, its formaton of thromboxane remains inhibited for the time the platelet remains in circulation (about 10 days). COX inhibition in other tissues is shorter due to resynthesis of new COX enzyme. Second, platelets almost completely express the COX-1 isoform which is about 100-fold more sensitive for ASA compared with COX-2.

An important difference between the anti-platelet activity of ASA and other NSAIDs is that ASA acts as an irreversible covalent inhibitor. As outlined above, NSAIDs bind to specific amino acids in the hydrophobic channel of COX enzymes in a noncovalent, reversible manner mediated by hydrogen bonds, polar and hydrophobic interaction. Therefore, COX inhibiton by non-aspirin NSAIDs is reversible, although there are differences between NSAIDs in the rate of recovery of COX activity after drug removal.

1.5 Drug/drug interactions between NSAIDs and aspirin

Clinically used doses of ASA have been titrated down to "low dose" (usually 70-100 mg/day) during the past decades to minimize side effects. However, this made ASA vulnerable for pharmacodynamic interactions with NSAIDs.

NSAIDs share the same pharmacological target as ASA, but they are not useful for platelet inhibition due to their reversible mode of action, which does not allow permanent complete platelet inhibition. Similarly, low dose ASA is inappropriate for anti-inflammatory treatment. Thus, low-dose ASA often must be coadministered with various NSAIDs in patients with cardiovascular and inflammatory rheumatic disease. There is a frequent co-morbidity of rheumatic and cardiovascular disease[30].

Unfortunately, NSAIDs may attenuate or even prevent platelet inhibtion by ASA by competing with ASA for access to the catalytic site of platelet COX-1. This has been suggested by several clinical studies either in vivo or in vitro for ibuprofen[31], naproxen[32,33] and others [27,34,35,36,37]. Since the cessation of antiplatelet therapy with ASA may substantially increase atherothombotic events and impair clinical outcome in patients with cardiovascular disease[38,39,40,41], a compromised pharmacodynamic action of ASA due to such drug/drug interactions is clinically important.

Some studies also suggested differences among individual NSAIDs with respect to their potential to interfere with low-dose ASA. For example, Catella-Lawson observed in healthy volunteers that ibuprofen, but not diclofenac, affect the antiplatelet effect of ASA[27]. This was later confirmed by Schuijt and coworkers[42]. Conflicting data exist for celecoxib, for which an interaction with ASA has been shown in vitro while it did not interfere with low-dose ASA in patients with osteoarthritis[43].

Unfortunately, it is still not entirely clear if this applies to single compounds or rather is a class effect of all NSAIDs. Therefore, an in vitro study is needed which compares a comprehensive selection of many individual NSAIDs, representative for all chemical groups of NSAID analgesics and examines their potential to interfere with the inhibition of platelet function by ASA.

To better understand the pharmacodynamic nature of this interaction, the present study examined platelet thromboxane formation, the mechanism of platelet activation targeted by ASA. Further, the molecular interaction between ASA and these NSAIDs in silico was examined by molecular docking studies.

1.6 Computer aided molecular docking, molecular design and Quantitative structural activity relationship (QSAR)

Computer assisted molecular design (CAMD) is a new technique which is used to accurately show the molecular reality, pharmacodynamic and pharmacokinetic properties of the molecules. It is widely used in field of pharmaceutical medicinal chemistry and pharmacy. Various parameters such as computation of binding free energies, empirical molecular mechanics, quantum mechanics, biological activity and molecular dynamics are used to study and design a new compound[44-47].

Molecular Docking

The main application of molecular docking is to study ligand or substrate binding. A number of docking programs are available which are based on different algorithms. According to mathematics, the conformation of ligand and receptor should be explored in six degrees of translational and rotational freedom. However, this is not possible in practice due to the size of the search space. CAMD can only detect a small amount of total conformational space. This is the major limitation of this technique. Mathematical constraints, restraints and approximations may overcome this problem to some degree. DOCK[48] is the pioneer software in which the docking algorithm was based on treating both ligand and target as rigid bodies. This software explored only six degrees of translational and rotational freedom.

CAMD field uses the following methods and techniques:

Molecular dynamics (MD): AUTODOCK[49] is a very commonly used docking program, which is based on MD method.

Monte Carlo (MC) methods: Monte Carlo method is one of the most widely used stochastic optimization techniques. AUTODOCK[49] and ICM (Internal Coordinates Mechanics)[50] softwares are good examples of programs using the MC method.

Genetic algorithms (GA) based methods: The essence of GA is the evolution of a population of possible solutions via genetic operators (mutations, crossovers and migrations) to a final population, optimizing a predefined fitness function. GOLD[51] and AUTODOCK[49] software programs are good examples of programs using this method.

Fragment based methods: In these methods the ligand is broken into separate portions or fragments, followed by docking the fragments and finally the fragments are joined together. An example of software using this method is FlexX[52].

Point complementarity methods: Complementarity properties between protein and ligand are also used to dock a ligand into protein. It differs from the fragment based methods because here the ligand is used as complete entity in its docking. FTDOCK50[53] and SANDOCK[54].

Distance geometry methods: Distance geometry methods determine the binding modes between protein and ligand considering only hydrogen bonding.

QSAR

QSAR originated in 19th century. Quantifying the relationship between structure and activity provides an understanding of the effect of structure of the drug on its pharmacokinetic or pharmacodynamic activity. The results of QSAR models can be used to understand the interactions between functional groups in molecules of greatest activity, with those of their target. QSAR is based on biological data, which naturally are subject to experimental variation and may be influenced by laboratory and environmental conditions. Hence, QSAR results predict the drug activity with limited precision.

In 1868, Crum-Brown and Fraser[55] published an equation, which is considered to be the first general equation of QSAR. They put forward the suggestion that physiological activity Φ of a series of quaternized strychnine derivatives depends on constitution (c), and suggested the following mathematical equation- (1)

$$\Phi = f(c) \qquad (1)$$

Meyer[56], Overton[57] and Ferguson[58] later applied the above principle and attempted the correlation of narcotic potencies with partition coefficient and thermodynamic parameters.

Hammet[59] in 1937 expressed the chemical reactivity of *meta*- and *para*-substituted benzene derivatives by eq. (2), where K_H is the rate constant for the parent (unsubstituted) molecule and K_x is the rate constant for the derivative.

$$\log(K_x/K_H) = \rho\sigma_x \quad (2)$$

The substitution constant σ_x refers to the electronic effect (potential) of the substituent relative to hydrogen. This is a parameter applicable to many different types of reactions characterized by different ρ values, whose relative rates depend on the electron donating or withdrawing power of the substituent. Since σ is defined in terms of ionization constants which can be related to free energies (ΔG) through equation (3), eq. (2) or any of its transformations can be considered as a linear free energy relationship (LFER).

$$\Delta G = -RT\ln K \quad (3)$$

Statistical Methods used in QSAR Analysis
Statistical methods play a key role in development of QSAR model[60-64]. Data analysis recombines data into forms and groups, observations into hierarchies. An often used statistical method is regression analysis.

1.7 Aims of the study

Based on the aforementioned techniques, it may be possible to examine the drug/drug interaction of ASA with NSAIDs experimentally and on a molecular level to elucidate several open questions. The following three major aims were addressed:

1. To study the molecular mechanism of drug interaction between ASA and NSAIDs by in silico docking.
2. To develop a QSAR model of this interaction in order to characterize factors which distinguish NSAIDs with respect to their propensitiy for interfering with ASA.
3. To examine whether the predictions of molecular modeling may correlate with experimental results that simulate the ASA/NSAID interaction in vitro.

2. MATERIALS AND METHODS

2.1 Drugs and chemicals

The study protocol used for the in vitro experiments was in agreement with the actual version of the declaration of Helsinki and approved by the University Düsseldorf Ethics committee (file No. 3205). A written informed consent was obtained from all voluntary blood donors. All subjects were healthy and negated to have taken any aspirin or other NSAIDs within 7 days before blood collection.

Selection of studied NSAID compounds:
In order to study the effect of NSAIDs on the anti-platelet activity of ASA, 22 widely used NSAIDs were selected, representing various chemical classes of NSAIDs as shown in table 3. Representatives of both frequently used and less frequently used NSAIDs were included. Among the most commonly prescribed NSAID compounds are the propionic acid derivatives ibuprofen and naproxen. Another popular group are the acetic acid derivatives, where diclofenac and indomethacin were selected. Since these are the leading NSAID classes, we included two representative compounds for each class. Less frequently used categories of NSAIDs are fenamates, oxicams, pyrazolinones and coxibs, of which we included flufenamate, piroxicam, dipyrone (active metabolite) and celecoxib. Celecoxib was chosen because it has some inhibitory activity on COX-1, other than rofecoxib or etoricoxib, which have higher COX-2 selectivity and, according to preliminary experiments, do not interfere with ASA. Celecoxib has recently been shown to interfere with ASA[65,66]. We also included nimesulide because it has some clinical importance as replacement for other NSAIDs in case of drug allergy.

ASA was used as its water soluble lysine salt (Aspirin i.v., Bayer, Leverkusen). Arachidonic acid was bought from Nu-Chek (Elysian, MN, USA) and transferred into the sodium salt before use. The sources of NSAIDs are given in table 3.

Table 3: Chemical category, individual compound and supplier of the NSAID compounds included in the study

Chemical class	Compound	Source
Heteroaryl acetic acids	Diclofenac,	Sigma-Aldrich, Deisenhofen
	Ketorolac	Sigma-Aldrich, Deisenhofen
	Sulindac	Sigma-Aldrich, Deisenhofen
	Nabumetone	Sigma-Aldrich, Deisenhofen
	6-MNA (*)	Cayman, US
	Indomethacin	Sigma-Aldrich, Deisenhofen
Propionic acids	S+ - Ibuprofen	Dolorgiet, St. Augustin
	Naproxen	Sigma-Aldrich, Deisenhofen
	Oxaprozin	Sigma-Aldrich, Deisenhofen
	Fenoprofen	Sigma-Aldrich, Deisenhofen
	Flurbiprofen	Sigma-Aldrich, Deisenhofen
	S+ - Ketoprofen	Sigma-Aldrich, Deisenhofen
Anthranilic acid	Flufenamic acid	Sigma-Aldrich, Deisenhofen
Enolic acids	Piroxicam	CT-Arzneimittel, Berlin
Sulphon derivative	Nimesulide	Sigma-Aldrich, Deisenhofen
Coxib	Celecoxib	Pfizer, Karlsruhe
Para-aminophenol	Acetaminophen (Paracetamol)	Sigma-Aldrich, Deisenhofen
Pyrazolinones	Methyl amino antipyrine (MAA**)	Prof. Dr. Weber
	Propyphenazone	Prof. Dr. Weber
	Phenazone	Prof. Dr. Weber
Fenamic acid derivative (Fenamates)	Mefenamic acid	Sigma-Aldrich, Deisenhofen
Acetic acid derivatives	Sulindac	Sigma-Aldrich, Deisenhofen
Arylalkonic acids	Tolmetin	Sigma-Aldrich, Deisenhofen

*) active metabolite of nabumetone, **) active metabolite of dipyrone
The pyrazolinone compounds were kindly provided by Prof. Dr. Horst Weber, Institut für Pharmazeutische Chemie, HHU Düsseldorf

2.2 Platelet aggregation and thromboxane formation

Venous blood was collected from healthy individuals into citrated (3.8%) vacutainers. Platelet counts were estimated in all collected samples and were always $\geq 100\,000$ µ/L.

Platelet rich plasma (PRP) was prepared by differential centrifugation after 30 min of blood collection. This included centrifugation of citrated (129 mmol/L) whole blood at 1400 rpm (10 min) in vacutainer tubes (10 mL) at room temperature (Labofuge, Heraeus Christ, Osterode). After centrufugation, PRP was collected using a plastic pipette and the pH corrected to pH 7.4 by careful addition of 1 mol/L NaOH or HCl. A small aliquot of platelet poor plasma was prepared by re-centrifugation of 5 mL of PRP at 2400 rpm for 10 min.

One mmol/L arachidonic acid was used to stimulate PRP aggregation, which was measured turbidimetrically on an APACT aggregometer at 37 °C (Labor, Hamburg, Germany). Aggregation measurements were started by addition of 250 µL PRP and 200 µL (Tyrode buffer) into micro cuvettes (Labor, Hamburg) pre-warmed at 37°C. After 2 min, the magnetic stirrer was started at 1000 rpm and the samples stirred for 2 additional min. Then, aspirin (30 µmol/L) or Tyrode buffer were added as appropriate. In order to examine the interference of selected NSAIDs with ASA, the NSAIDs were added at the same time as ASA. The final volume of aggregation was always 500 µL. ASA with or without NSAIDs was incubated in PRP for additional 5 min (separate experiments with longer times of pre-incubation with NSAIDs obtained identical results). Thereafter, arachidonic acid (1 mmol/L) (Nu-Chek, Elysian, MN, USA) was added to induce platelet aggregation, which was recorded for 4 min. Finally, platelet suspensions were centrifuged at 14000 x g for 5 min and the supernatants were used to determine platelet thromboxane formation (TXB_2) by radioimmunoassay. Aggregation was expressed as maximum change in light transmission (cm min^{-1} recorder deflection).

To determine TXB_2 in the supernatants obtained after aggregation, the samples were diluted 1/1000 by sodium phosphate buffer (150mM NaCl; 8mM Na_2HPO_4 x H_2O; 1,7mM NaH_2PO_4 x $2H_2O$; pH 7,4) and 750µL aliquots further processed by addition of 20 pg radioactive tracer ($3HTXB_2$, Perkin Elmer, Frankfurt). Antiserum (rabbit, own production) was added at 1/5000 and the samples were allowed to sit for 20 h at room temperature. Then bound activity was separated from free by adding 500 µl of charcoal/dextrane 500 (25%/2.5%) suspension. One ml aliquots of these supernatants were counted in 10 ml of scintillator counter (Lumasafe Plus, Perkin Elmer, USA). Plasma TXB_2 concentrations were calculated by a linearized calibration curve. For standardization, the obtained TXB_2 concentrations were calculated as % of control samples without ASA and without the respective NSAIDs.

2.3 Molecular modeling and docking studies

MolDock is a docking module of Molegro Virtual Docker (MVD) software[67]. It is based on a new hybrid search algorithm, called guided differential evolution (DE). The guided DE algorithm combines the differential evolution optimization techniques with a cavity prediction algorithm. DE was introduced by Storn and Price in 1995 and has previously been successfully applied to molecular docking[68]. The use of predicted cavities during the search process allows for a fast and accurate identification of potential binding modes (poses). The docking scoring function of MolDock is based on a piecewise linear potential (PLP) introduced by Gehlhaar et al[69-71]. In MolDock, the docking scoring function is extended with a new term, taking hydrogen bond directionality into account. Moreover, a re-ranking procedure is applied to the highest ranked poses to further increase the docking accuracy.

This automatic docking software, Molegro Virtual Docker, was used in the present docking studies. The reported crystal structure of COX-I[72] (PDB ID:1PGG)[73] was downloaded from Brookhaven Protein Data Bank (PDB) for the purpose of docking studies. Initially, the protein was considered without ligand and water molecules. The backbone was fixed, the CharmM force field and minimization using steep descent algorithm was applied for the protein (COX-I). All the NSAIDs were prepared using the CharmM force field and minimized up to a gradient of 0.01 kcal (mol Å)$^{-1}$ with help of Discovery Studio 2.0 software[74].

Due to the availability of the co-crystallized ligand PGHS-iodoindomethacin (PDB ID: 1PGG)[73], we used the template docking available in the Molegro virtual docker and evaluated the MolDock, rerank and protein - ligand interaction scores from MolDock [GRID] options. Template docking is based on extracting the chemical properties like the pharmacophore elements of a ligand bound in the active site. This information is utilized in the docking of the structurally similar analogs. The iodoindomethacin from 1PGG was used as the template with the default settings, including a grid resolution of 0.30, for grid generation and a 11 Å radius from the template as the binding site. The MolDock SE was used as a search algorithm, and the number of runs was set to 10. A population size of 50, maximum iteration of 1500 for parameter settings was used. The maximum number of poses to generate was 10. Since the Molegro virtual docker works by an evolutionary algorithm, consecutive docking runs do not give exactly the same pose and interactions. To address this issue of inherent randomness, three consecutive runs were done and the top three poses were used to visualize the interactions of the selected NSAIDs. Validation of the docking was done by comparing the docked posed of flurbiprofen with its X ray crystal structure from database ((PDB ID: 1CQE)[75]. The chemical structures used for the molecular docking were obtained from pubchem database. These structures are shown in table 4.

Table 4: Structures obtained from PubChem database used for docking analysis

Acetaminophen	Celecoxib	Diclofenac
Dipyrone (Metamizol)	Flurbiprofen	Fenoprofen
Flufenamic acid	(S+)Ibuprofen	Indomethacin

Ketoprofen	Ketorolac	MAA
Mefenamic acid	6- MNA (6 Methoxy 2 napthalene acetic acid)	Nabumetone
Naproxen	Nimesulide	NS-398
Oxaprozin	Phenazone	Piroxicam
Propyphenazone	Sulinidac sulfide	Tolmentin

2.4 Mathematical modeling (QSAR)

The concentration (μmol/L) of NSAIDs, showing interaction with ASA, required for 25 % increase in the platelet aggregation and TXB_2 activity, respectively, was determined from the in-vitro experiments using linear regression. The mathematical modeling was based on the correlation of IC_{50} and selectivity of NSAIDs towards COX-I over COX-II enzyme. IC_{50} values for NSAIDs towards COX-I and COX-II were obtained from literature[76] and selectivity ratios (IC_{50} for COX-I/ IC_{50} for COX-II) were calculated for all NSAIDs. Those NSAIDs, where IC_{50} values were not documented for both COX isoforms, could not be used for QSAR analysis. Linear and non-linear regression was performed and the correlation coefficient was calculated using SYSTAT software[77].

The following different types of regression analysis were used to develop a mathematical model:

- Simple linear regression analysis: An independent variable is correlated with a dependent variable and produces a linear one-term equation.
- Multiple linear regression analysis (MLR): More than one independent variable is correlated with dependent variable and a single multi term equation is formed.
- Stepwise linear regression analysis: The number of independent variables is high and is thus correlated in a stepwise manner with the dependent variable, producing a multi term linear equation.

The following definitions of mathematical terms have been used in our QSAR model:

(a) Correlation Coefficient (r): The correlation coefficient r is a measure of the quality of the fit of the model because its value depends on the overall variance of the dependent variable.

$r = \sqrt{1 - \sum \Delta^2 / S_{yy}}$ (Eq^n-1)

Where, S_{yy} is overall variance i.e $S_{yy} = \sum(y_{obs} - y_{mean})^2$; $\sum \Delta^2 = SSQ - \sum(y_{obs} - y_{cal})^2$; '$y_{obs}$' and '$y_{calc}$' are observed and calculated biological activities, 'y_{mean}' is mean of biological activities.

(b) Square of the Correlation Coefficient (Coefficient of Determination, r^2)

The squared correlation r^2 is a measure of the explained variance, most often presented as a percentage value e.g. $r^2=0.664$ as 66.4%.

$r2 = 1-\sum\Delta^2/Syy$ (Eq^n-2)

(c) Standard Deviation (SD)

This is a measure of how well the function derived by the QSAR analysis predicts the observed biological activity. Its value considers the number of object 'n' and the number of variable 'k'. Therefore, SD depends not only on the quality of fit but also on the number of degrees of freedom (DF). The smaller the value of SD the better is the QSAR model.

$DF = n-k-1; SD = \sqrt{\sum(y_{obs} - y_{cal})^2 / n-k-1}$ (Eq^n-3)

(e) Cross-validation r^2 (r^2_{cv}, or q^2)

Cross-validation is an approach for selecting a model which is most likely to have predictive value. This proceeds by omitting one or more rows of input data, re-deriving the model, and predicting the target property values of the omitted rows. The re-derivation and predicting cycle continues till all target property values have been predicted at least once. The root mean square error of all target predictions, the PRESS (predictive sum of squares) is the basis for evaluating the model. This is obtained using following formula,

$r^2_{cv} = [SD-PRESS]/SD$,   (Eq^n-5)

where SD is standard deviation. A cross-validated r^2 is usually smaller than the overall r^2 for a QSAR equation.

2.5 Statistical evaluation of the experimental results

All data represent mean values ± SEM of n observations. Comparisons between groups were performed using the ANOVA on ranks for repeated measures. Post hoc analyses for differences between groups were performed by Dunnet's test.

P values < 0.05 were considered statistically significant. Comparision between 2 groups was done Wilcoxon U test.

3. RESULTS

3.1 Experimental results

NSAID interaction with aspirin-induced inhibition of platelet function

Platelet aggregation in control samples of platelet rich plasma without addition of COX inhibitors ranged from 14 to 20 cm min^{-1}. 30 µmol/ L ASA completely inhibited platelet aggregation in all samples when NSAIDs were not present.

However, the majority of the studied NSAIDs markedly altered the inhibition of aggregation by ASA. For example, when ASA (30 µmol/L) was added together with ibuprofen (10 µmol/L), there was a strong aggregation suggesting that ibuprofen potently interfered with the platelet inhibitory action of ASA (figure 2e). Several other NSAIDs interfered with 30 µmol/L ASA similar as ibuprofen (figure 2e). These were celecoxib, fenoprofen, flufenamic acid, mefenamic acid, nabumetone, naproxen, nimesulide, oxaprozin , phenazone, piroxicam, propyphenazone, sulindac, tolmetin and 6 -MNA. Fenoprofen, flufenamic and mefenamic acid, nabumetone, nimesulide, tolmetin and 6-MNA almost completely abolished platelet inhibition by ASA. The maximum aggregation observed in presence of ASA (30 µmol/L) plus one of these NSAIDs were not significantly different from control (paired t-test, $p>0.05$).

In contrast, ibuprofen, naproxen, celecoxib, methylaminoantipyrine (the active metabolite of dipyrone), oxaprozin, phenazone, piroxicam, propyphenazone, sulindac appeared to less potently attenuate inhibition by ASA. This was indicated by the fact that aggregation remained significantly below control at all concentrations of these NSAIDs (paired t-test, $p<0.05$). Interestingly, the concentration-response curves of celecoxib, dipyrone, nabumetone, naproxen, nimesulide, oxaprozin, propyphenazone, sulindac, tolmetin and 6-MNA showed a decline of aggregation at their highest concentrations (figure 2).

In contrast to the aforementioned NSAIDs, acetaminophen, diclofenac, flurbiprofen, indomethacin, ketoprofen and ketorolac did not interfere with ASA at all and aggregation remained completely inhibited even if the concentrations of these inhibitors were raised up to a high micromolar range (figure 3).

NSAID interaction with aspirin-induced inhibition of platelet TXB_2 formation

TXB_2 formation in control samples without addition of COX inhibitors was 2005 ± 109 ng mL-1 and was set 100 % in order to express the relative inhibition of COX activity by ASA in vitro. 30 µmol/L ASA (without NSAID) inhibited TXB_2 formation to less than 5% (84 ± 7 ng mL-1, $p<0.05$ for all NSAID compounds).

Several NSAIDs partially or completely prevented this inhibition. For example, when 10 µmol/L ibuprofen and 30 µmol/L ASA were added together, platelet TXB_2 formation was 456 ± 135 ng mL^{-1} ($p<0.05$ vs. control). Hence, ibuprofen interfered with ASA-induced inhibition of thromboxane formation similar as observed for aggregation.

Moreover, celecoxib, fenoprofen, flufenamic acid, mefenamic acid, methylamino-antipyrine, nabumetone, naproxen, nimesulide, oxaprozin, piroxicam, propyphenazone, phenazone, sulindac, tolmetin and 6-MNA also interfered with the inhibition of TXB_2 formation by ASA. The concentration-response curves of some NSAIDs declined at the highest concentration studied in a similar manner as observed for aggregation.

In contrast, acetaminophen, diclofenac, flurbiprofen, indomethacin, ketoprofen, and ketorolac did not interfere with aspirin with respect to inhibition of platelet TXB_2 synthesis. Diclofenac inhibited TXB_2 biosynthesis synergistically with aspirin and this inhibition reached statistical significance (figure 3).

Figure 2 (next pages): NSAIDs showing interaction with ASA-induced inhibition of platelet aggregation (right graph) and platelet TXB2 formation (left graph). Each graph shows the inhibition of TXB2 formation or aggregation by ASA (30 µmol/L) alone (bars) and concentration-dependent effect of NSAIDs on inhibition by ASA(30 µmol/L) (line graph). Asterisks denote significant differences from ASA alone ($p<0.05$).

(a) Celecoxib:

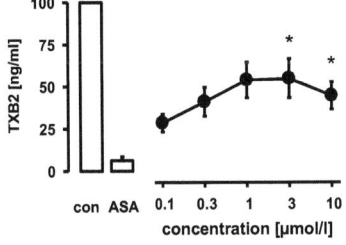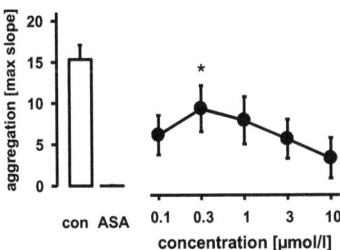

(b) **Methylaminoantipyrine:**

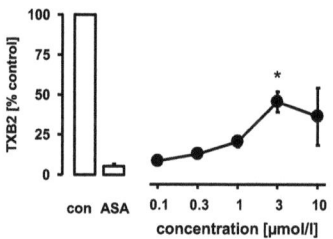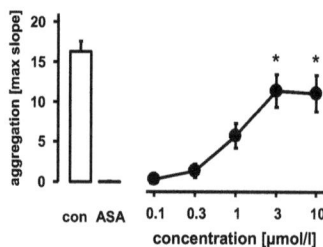

(c) **Fenoprofen:**

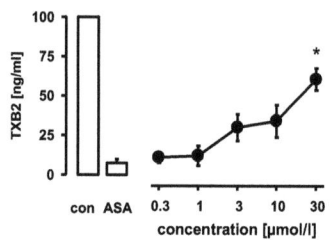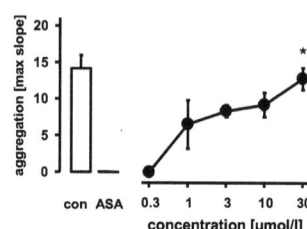

(d) **Flufenamic acid:**

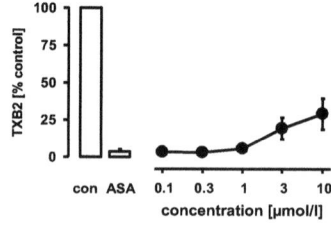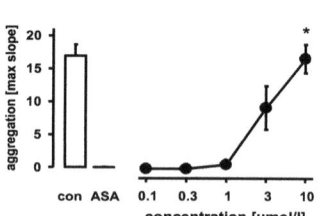

(e) **Ibuprofen:**

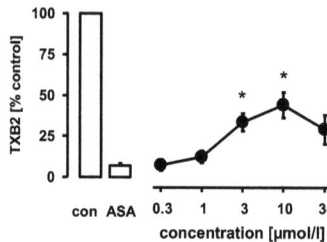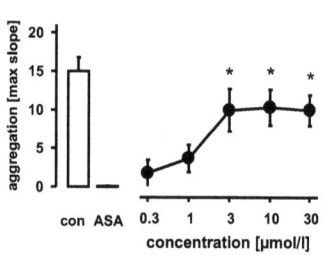

(f) **Mefenamic acid:**

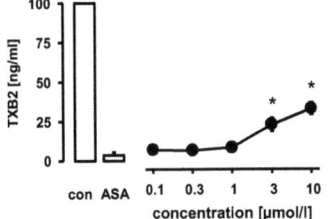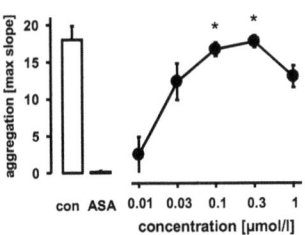

(g) **Nabumetone:**

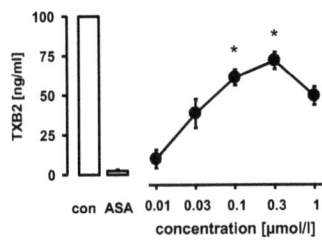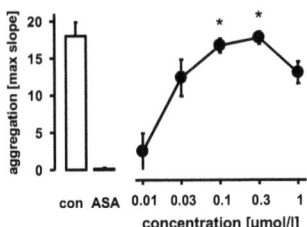

(h) **Naproxen**

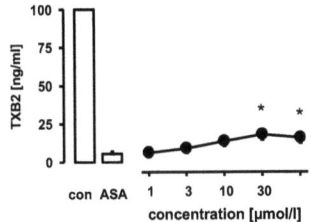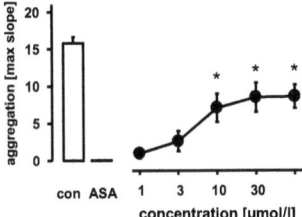

(i) **Nimesulide:**

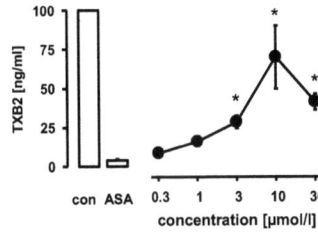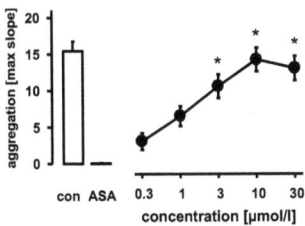

(j) **Oxaprozin:**

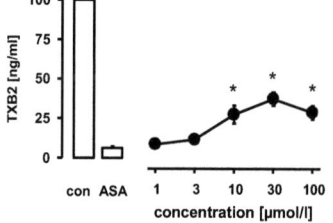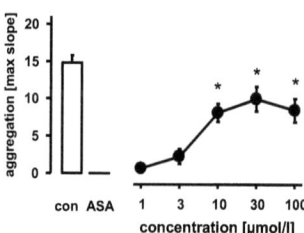

(k) **Phenazone:**

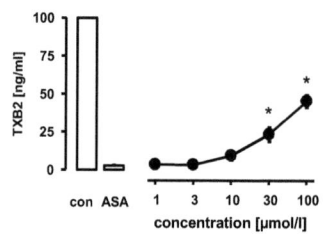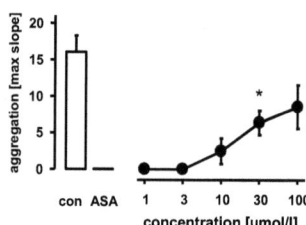

(l) **Piroxicam:**

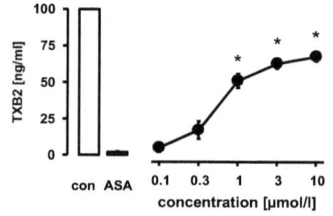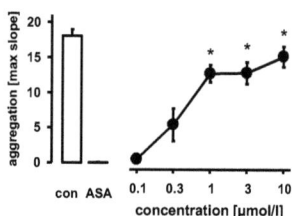

(m) Propyphenazone:

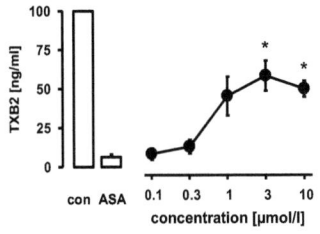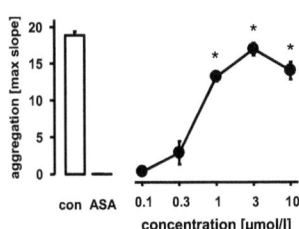

(n) Sulindac sulfide:

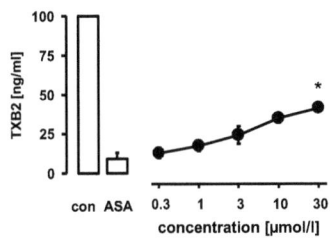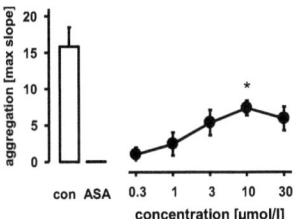

(o) Tolmetin:

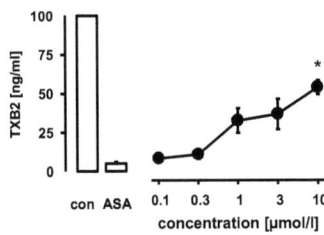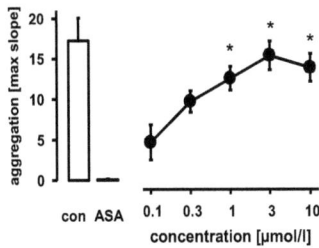

(p) 6-MNA:

Figure 3 (next pages): NSAIDs not showing interaction with ASA-induced inhibition of platelet function and platelet TXB2 formation. For further explanation see legend of figure 2

(a) Acetaminophen:

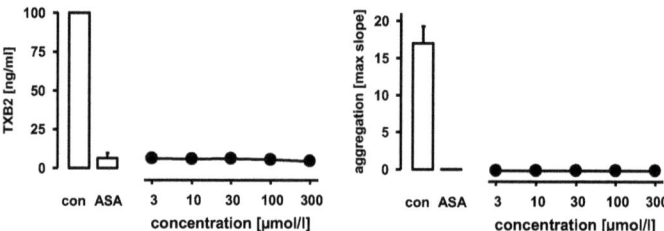

(b) Diclofenac:

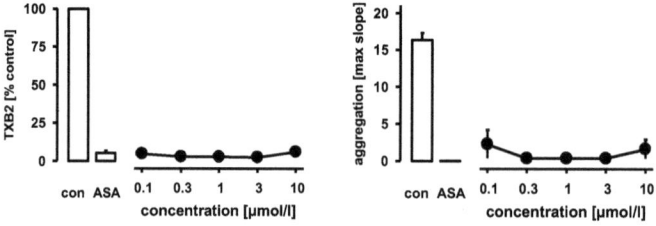

(c) Flurbiprofen:

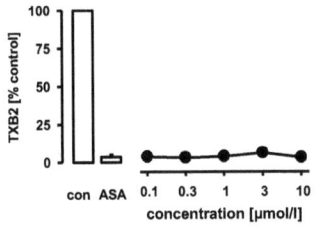
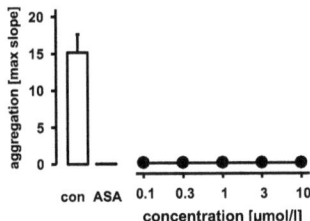

(d) Indomethacin:

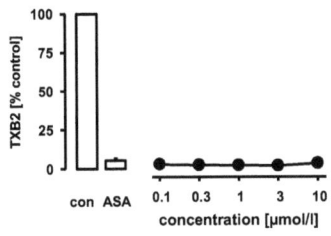
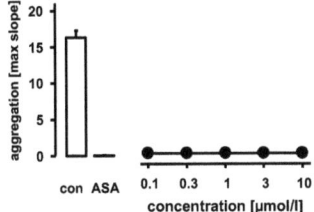

(e) Ketoprofen:

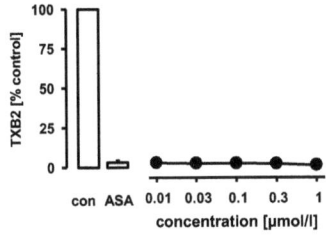
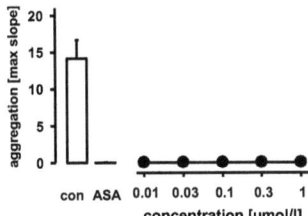

(f) Ketorolac:

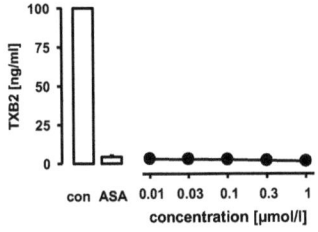
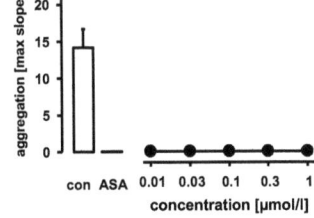

3.2 QSAR results

On the basis of experimental results, QSAR studies were performed in order to predict the factors on which antiplatelet activity of ASA might be dependent in presence of a particular NSAID.

The concentration (conc.) of NSAID required for 25% increase in the platelet aggregation and in the TXB_2 formation were determined from the in vitro experiments.

IC_{50} values for all NSAIDs for COX-I and COX-II respectively, were obtained from one research publication[76], which determined this parameter by an identical methodology. COX-I/COX-II selectivity of a particular NSAID was calculated on the basis of NSAID's IC_{50} values for COX-I and COX-II and is shown in table 5.

Table 5: Parameters used for QSAR model development:

Comp. No.	Drugs	Conc. (µmol/L) of NSAIDs for 25 % increase in platelet aggregation	Conc. (µmol/L) of NSAIDs for 25% increase in TXB_2 formation	IC_{50} (µmol/L) COX-I	IC_{50} (µmol/L) COX-II	Selectivity COX-I/II
1	Celecoxib	0.01	2.03	NA	NA	NA
2	Dipyrone	0.18	1.27	NA	NA	NA
3	Fenoprofen	0.09	0.71	2.73	14.03	0.19
4	Flufenamic acid	1.58	5.37	NA	NA	NA
5	Ibuprofen	0.57	6.44	5.9	9.9	0.59
6	Mefenamic acid	1.71	4.35	1.94	0.16	12.1
7	Nabumetone	13.26	34.38	33.57	20.83	1.61
8	Naproxen	NA	NA	32.01	28.19	1.14
9	Nimesulide	0.045	2.03	10.48	0.18	58.22
10	Oxaprozin	6.38	11.47	14.58	36.67	0.40
11	Phenazone	18.94	34.38	NA	NA	NA
12	Piroxicam	0.29	0.45	2.68	2.11	1.27
13	Propylphenazone	0.11	0.52	NA	NA	NA
14	Sulindac Sulfide	3.27	3.51	NA	NA	NA
15	Tolmetin	0.092	0.71	1.08	2.25	0.48
16	6-MNA	10.99	44.37	31.01	19.84	1.56
17	Aspirin	NA	NA	4.45	13.88	0.32
18	Acetaminophen	No effect	No effect	42.23	10.69	4
19	Indomethacin	No effect	No effect	0.21	0.37	0.56
20	Diclofenac	No effect	No effect	0.26	0.01	26
21	Flurbiprofen	No effect	No effect	0.41	4.23	0.1
22	Ketoprofen	No effect	No effect	0.11	0.88	0.12

Regression analysis was performed among the parameters mentioned in table 5 and figure 4-8 were obtained.

Figure 4 represents a plot between the concentration of a particular NSAID required for 25% increase in the platelet aggregation (x-axis) and 25% increase in the TXB2 formation (y-axis) in presence of aspirin for 15 NSAIDs which interfered with antiplatelet activity of aspirin in the in vitro experiments (section 3.1). These 15 NSAIDs included celecoxib, dipyrone, fenoprofen, flufenamic acid, ibuprofen, mefenamic acid, nabumetone, nimesulide, oxaprozin, phenazone, piroxicam, propylphenazone, sulindac sulfide, tolmetin and 6-MNA. Naproxen could not be included in the figure because a 25% increase in platelet aggregation and TXB_2 formation was not observed experimentally (see fig. 2h in of experimental results).

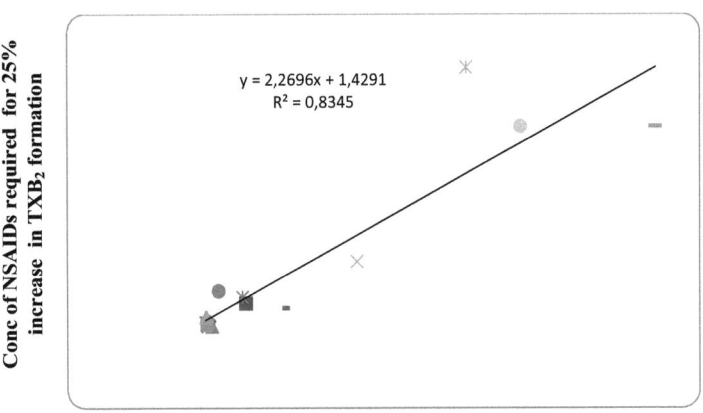

Conc. of NSAIDs required for 25% increase in platelet aggregation

Figure 5 (on next page) represents a plot between the concentration of 9 individual NSAIDs required for 25% increase in the platelet aggregation (x-axis) and the corresponding COX-I IC_{50} value (y-axis). Only 9 NSAIDs could be included here, because the COX-I IC_{50} values were available in publication[76] only for those 9 NSAIDs. These included fenoprofen, ibuprofen, mefenamic acid, nabumetone, nimesulide, oxaprozin, piroxicam, tolmetin and 6-MNA.

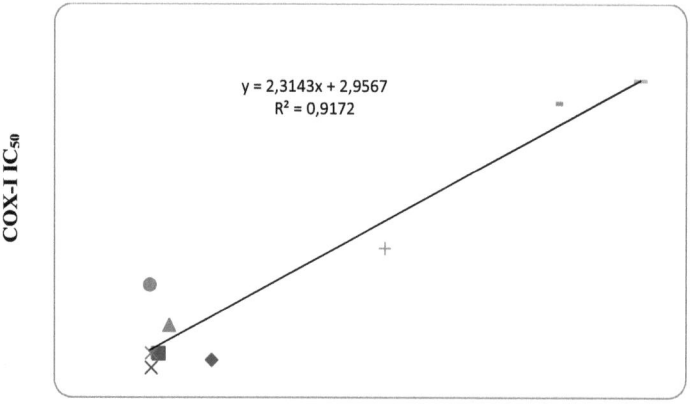

Conc. of NSAIDs required for 25% increase in platelet aggregation

Figure 6 Similarly, figure 6 represents a plot between the concentration of these NSAIDs required for 25% increase in platelet aggregation (x-axis) and their corresponding COX-II IC_{50} value. As in case of figure 5, figure 6 contains 9 NSAIDs because COX-II IC_{50} values were available only for fenoprofen, ibuprofen, mefenamic acid, nabumetone, nimesulide, oxaprozin, piroxicam, tolmetin and 6-MNA in the respective publication[76]. Fenoprofen and oxaprozin were considered as outliers in figure 6 shown below.

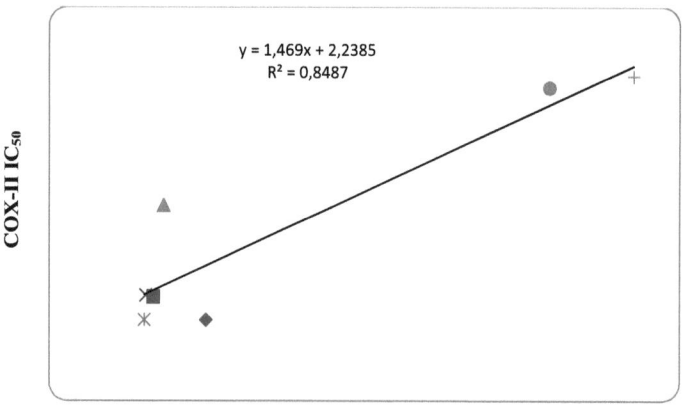

Conc. of NSAIDs required for 25% increase in platelet aggregation

Figure 7 represents the plot between the concentration of NSAID required for 25 % increase in the TXB_2 formation (x-axis) and its particular IC_{50} for COX-I (y-axis). Similarly to figure 5 and figure 6, figure 7 also includes fenoprofen, ibuprofen, mefenamic acid, nabumetone, nimesulide, oxaprozin, piroxicam, tolmetin and 6-MNA.

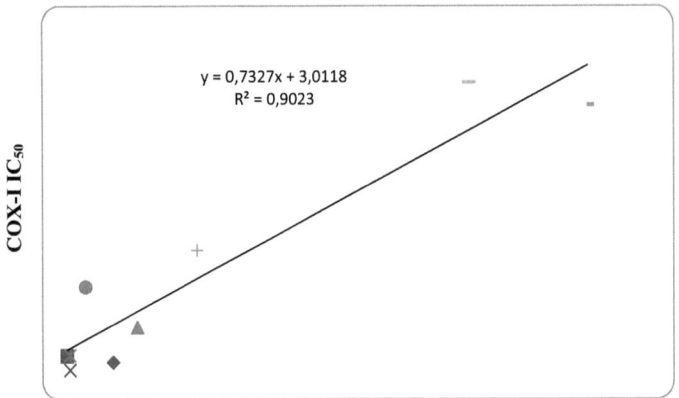

Conc. of NSAIDs required for 25% increase in TXB_2 formation

Figure 8(on next page) represents the plot between the NSAID concentration required for 25 % increase in TXB_2 formation (x-axis) and the respective IC_{50} for inhibition of COX-II (y-axis). Similarly to figure 5 ,6 and 7, figure 8 included ibuprofen, mefenamic acid, nabumetone, nimesulide, piroxicam, tolmetin and 6-MNA. Similar to figure 6, in figure 8 fenoprofen and oxaprozin were considered as outliers.

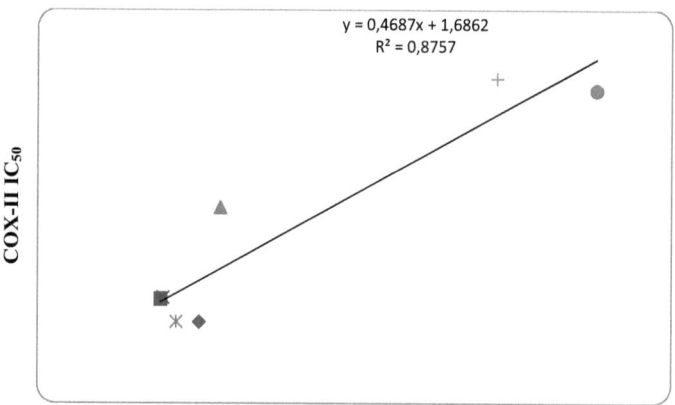

Conc. of NSAIDs required for 25% increase in TXB$_2$ formation

3.3 Docking results

Molegro virtual docking software was used to study hydrogen bond interaction of the drugs at the COX-I catalytic site. Template docking was done on reported crystal structure of COX-I (PDB ID:1PGG)[73] downloaded from Brookhaven Protein data Bank. The docking protocol used by Molegro was cross checked by perfoming docking studies of flurbiprofen in COX-I catalytic site and comparing it with the available crystal structure of flurbiprofen bound to human COX-I (PDB ID: 1CQE)[75] (see figure 9)

Figure 9 (on next page): The superimposition of best pose of flurbiprofen (green colour) with co-crystallized structure flurbiprofen (silver grey colour) from PDB ID: 1CQE in the active site of COX-I.

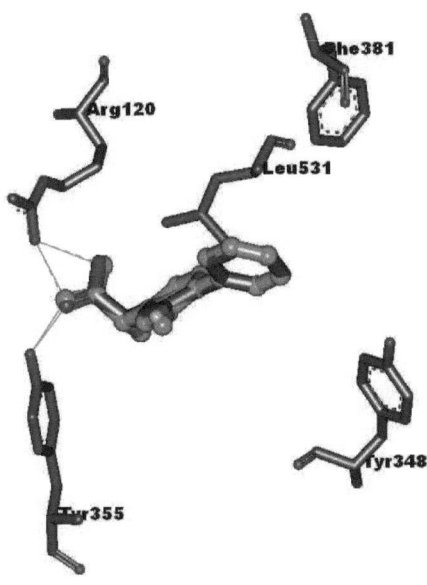

Naproxen, nimesulide, oxaprozin, flufenamic acid, piroxicam and dipyrone (MAA) were found to form hydrogen bonds with Ser 530, the target site for acetylation by aspirin. Active channel in COX-I comprises of Tyr 385, Ser 530, Arg 120, Tyr 355 and Trp 387 and hence docking of all selected NSAIDs were focused in the active channel in COX-I[20]. All these NSAIDs also interfered with the antiplatelet activity of aspirin in the in vitro experiments. However, hydrogen bond interactions with other amino acids in the hydrophobic channel were also seen. Celecoxib formed 2 hydrogen bond interactions with Arg 120 and Tyr 355. Ibuprofen also formed hydrogen bond interactions with Arg 120 and Tyr 355. Naproxen, nimesulide, oxaprozin, flufenamic acid, piroxicam and dipyrone (MAA) also formed at least two hydrogen bonds with either of Tyr 385, Arg 120, Tyr 355 or Ser 530 (see figure 10). All bond lengths as shown in table 6 were less than 3.5 Å[78], which is required for hydrogen bond interactions.

In contrast, NSAIDs which experimentally did not show any interference with anti-platelet activity of ASA (diclofenac, ketorolac and acetaminophen), also did not show any hydrogen bond interactions with Ser 530 and other relevant amino acids present in the hydrophobic active channel (see figure 11). No hydrogen bond interactions were reported in docking analysis of diclofenac and ketorolac. Acetaminophen showed only one hydrogen bond interaction with Arg 120.

Table 6: Results of NSAIDs docking in COXs-1 active channel. Bond lengths are represented in Amstrong (Å)

SN	Comp	TYR385 (Å)	SER530 (Å)	ARG120 (Å)	TYR355 (Å)	TRP387 (Å)	I Interference
a	Celecoxib	-	-	-	3.402	-	Y
b	Diyprone (Metamizol)	-	-	1(2.765)	1(2.593)	-	Y
c	Fenoprofen	-	-	2(3.193;3.172)	3.069	-	Y
d	Flufenamic acid	1(3.151)	1(2.755) Å	-	-	-	Y
e	Ibuprofen	1(2.017)	2(2.861;3.092)	-	-	-	Y
f	MAA	-	2(2.865;3.064)	-	-	-	Y
g	Mefenamic acid	1(2.759)	1(2.940)	-	-	-	Y
h	Nabumeton	1(2.763)	1(1.333)	-	-	-	Y
i	Naproxen	-	-	1(2.558)	1(2.757)	-	Y
j	Nimesulide	1(2,859)	2(2.632;2.623)	-	-	-	Y
k	NS 398	-	1(2,668)	-	-	-	Y
l	Oxaprozin	1(2.724)	2(2.754;3.185)	-	-	-	Y
m	Phenazone	1(2.651)	1(3.176)	-	-	-	Y
n	Piroxicam	1(2.711)	2(3.107;3.025)	-	-	-	Y
o	Propyphenazone	1(2.651)	1(2.597)	-	-	-	Y
p	Sulindac sulfide	-	-	1(2.517)	1(3.073)	-	Y
q	Tolmetin	-	-	2(2.856;2.835)	-	-	Y
r	Acetaminophen	-	-	1(2.980)	-	-	N
s	Diclofenac	-	-	-	-	-	N
t	Flurbiprofen	-	-	2(3.102;2.638)	1(2.839)	-	N
u	Indomethacin	-	-	2(2.336;2.466)	-	-	N
v	Ketoprofen	-	-	-	-	-	N
w	Ketorolac	-	-	-	-	-	N

Figure 10 a-q (on next page): Docking of NSAIDs which decreased the antiplatelet activity of ASA in *invitro* experiments. Atom type colour code: Carbon=grey, chlorine=green, fluorine=skyblue, nitrogen=blue, oxygen=red, sulfur=yellow.

a. Celecoxib

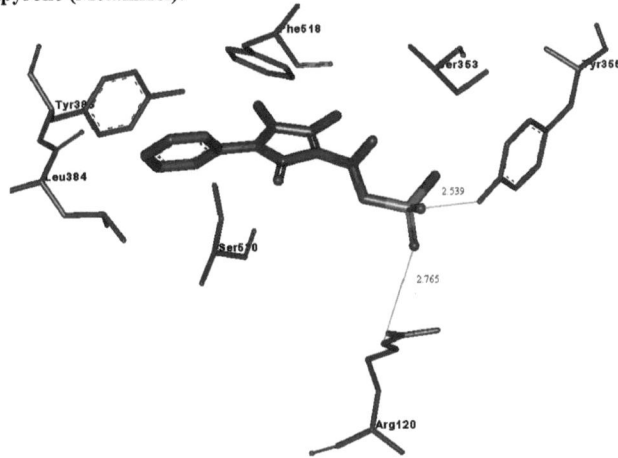

Celecoxib forms in total 4 hydrogen bond interaction, one with Tyr 355(BL = 3.402 Å), second one with Ser 516 (BL= 3.163 Å) , third one with Ile 517 (BL = 3.155 Å) and fourth one with Phe 518 (BL = 3.116 Å).A decrease in antiplatelet activity of ASA was seen in the presence of celecoxib in the invitro experiments.

b. Dipyrone (Metamizol):

Dipyrone forms 2 hydrogen bond interactions with Arg 120 (BL = 2.765 Å) & Tyr 355 (BL = 2.593 Å) respectively. A decrease in antiplatelet activity of ASA was seen in the presence of dipyrone in the invitro experiments.

c. Fenoprofen:

Fenoprofen forms 2 hydrogen bond interactions with Arg 120 having bond lengths 3.193 Å and 3.172 Å respectively. One hydrogen bond interaction with Tyr 355 (BL = 3.069 Å). There was a decrease of the antiplatelet activity of ASA in presence of fenoprofen in the in vitro experiments.

d. Flufenamic acid:

Flufenamic acid docking result showed that it forms one hydrogen bond interaction with Ser 530 (BL = 2.755 Å) and one hydrogen bond interaction with Tyr 385 (BL =

3.151 Å). A decrease in antiplatelet activity of ASA was seen in the presence of flufenamic acid in the invitro experiments.

e. Ibuprofen:

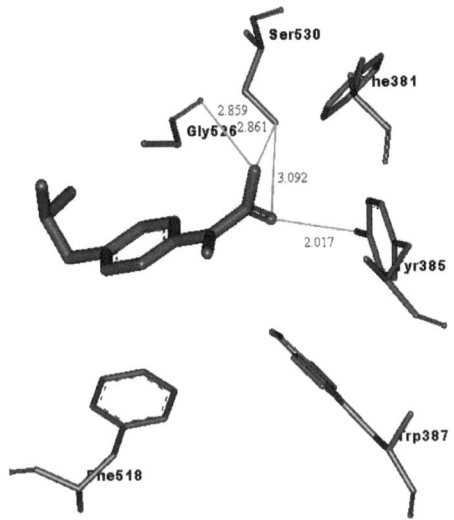

Ibuprofen forms two hydrogen bond interaction with Ser 530 (BL = 2.861 Å and BL = 3.092 Å), one hydrogen bond interaction with Tyr 385 (BL = 2.017 Å) and one hydrogen bond interaction with Gly 526 (BL = 2.859 Å). A decrease in antiplatelet activity of ASA was also seen in the presence of ibuprofen in the invitro experiments.

f. Methylaminoantipyrin:

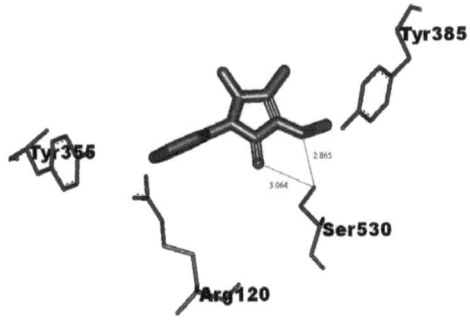

Methylaminoantipyrin, the active metabolite of dipyrone, forms 2 hydrogen bonds with Ser 530 (BL = 2.865 Å and BL = 3.064 Å). A decrease in antiplatelet activity of ASA was observed in the presence of MAA in the invitro experiments.

g. Mefenamic acid:

Mefenamic acid showed 2 hydrogen bond interaction with Ser 530 (BL = 2.940 Å) and Tyr 385 (BL = 2.759) Å respectively. A decrease in antiplatelet activity of ASA was observed in the presence of mefenamic acid in the invitro experiments.

h. Nabumeton:

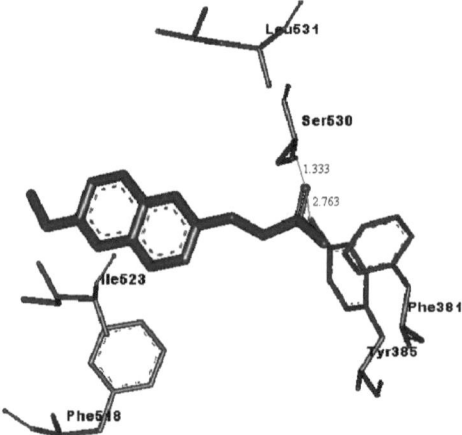

Nabumeton forms 2 hydrogen bonds with Tyr 385 (BL = 2.763 Å) and Ser 530 (BL= 1.333 Å) respectively. A decrease in antiplatelet activity of ASA was seen in the presence of Nabumeton in the invitro experiments.

i. Naproxen:

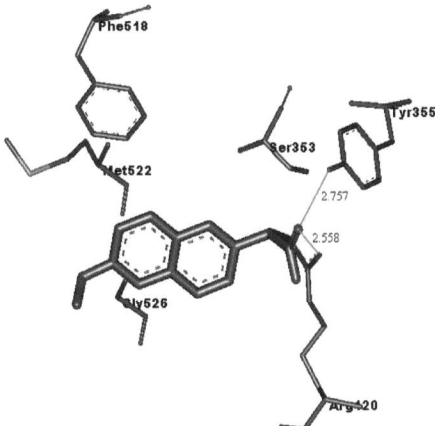

Naproxen forms 2 hydrogen bonds interactions. One with Tyr 355 (BL = 2.757 Å) and another one with Arg 120 (BL = 2.558 Å). A decrease in the antiplatelet activity of ASA was seen in the presence of naproxen in the invitro experiments.

j. Nimesulide:

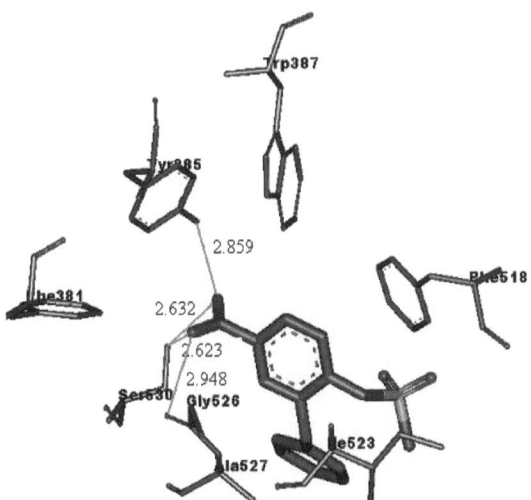

Nimesulide forms in total 4 hydrogen bond interactions. One hydrogen bond interaction with Tyr 385 (BL = 2.859 Å), two hydrogen bond interactions with Ser 530 (BL = 2,632 Å, BL = 2.623 Å) and one hydrogen bond interaction with Gly 526

(BL = 2.948 Å). A decrease in the antiplatelet activity of ASA was also seen in the presence of nimesulide in invitro experiments.

k. NS 398:

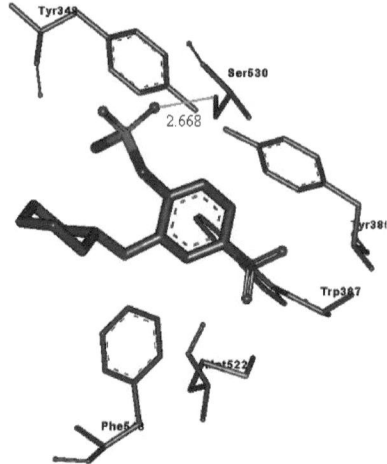

NS-398, a COX-2 preferential inhibitor with some activity on COX-1, forms only one hydrogen bond interaction with Ser 530 (BL = 2.668 Å) respectively. A decrease in the antiplatelet activity of ASA was seen in the presence of NS-398 in the invitro experiments.

l. Oxaprozin:

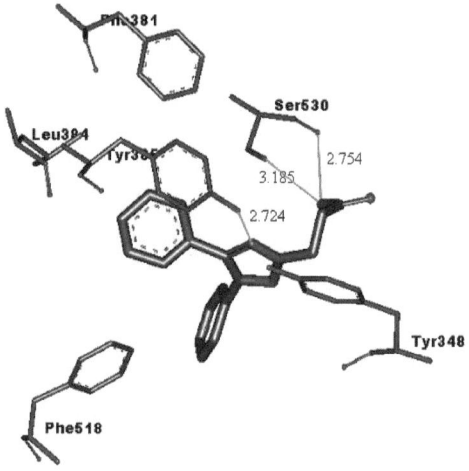

Oxaprozin forms two hydrogen bond interaction with Ser 530 (BL = 3.185 Å and BL = 2.754) and one hydrogen bond interaction with Try 385 (BL= 2.724 Å). A decrease in the antiplatelet activity of ASA was seen in the presence of oxaprozin in the invitro experiments.

m. Phenazone:

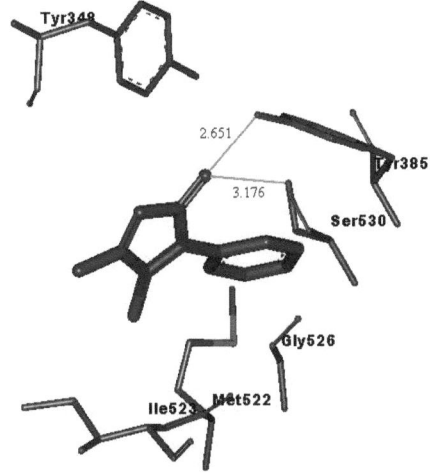

Phenazone, which is structurally related to MAA (above), forms one hydrogen bond interaction with Ser 530 (BL = 3.176 Å) and Tyr-385 (BL = 2.651 Å). A decrease in the antiplatelet activity of ASA was seen in the presence of phenazone in the in vitro experiments.

n. Piroxicam:

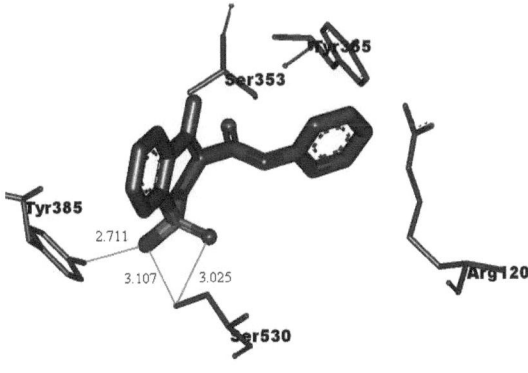

Piroxicam forms two hydrogen bond interactions with Ser 530 (BL = 3.025 Å and BL = 3.107 Å) and one hydrogen bond with Tyr 385 (BL = 2.711 Å). A decrease in antiplatelet activity of ASA was seen in presence of piroxicam in the in vitro experiments.

o. Propylphenazone:

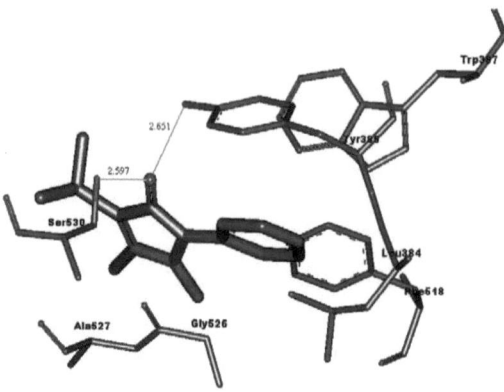

The docking results with propyphenazone showed one hydrogen bond interaction with Ser 530 (BL = 2.597 Å) and another one with Try 385 (BL = 2.651 Å). A decrease in the antiplatelet activity of ASA was seen in the presence of propyphenazone in the in vitro experiments.

p. Sulindac Sulfide:

Sulindac sulfide docking result showed one hydrogen bond interaction with Tyr 355 (BL = 3.073 Å) and one with Arg 120 (BL = 2.517 Å). A decrease in antiplatelet activity of ASA was seen in presence of sulindac in invitro experiment.

r. Tolmetin:

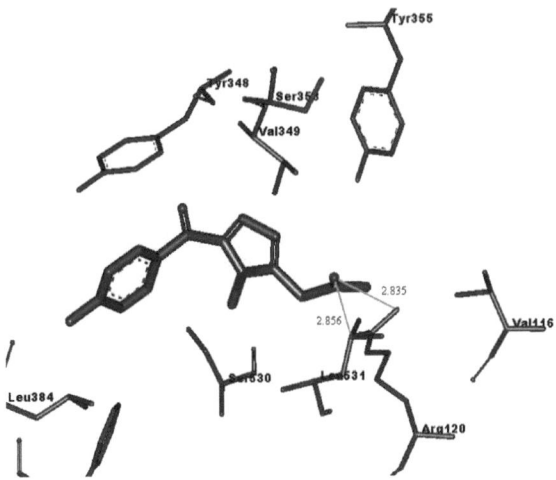

Tolmetin forms 2 hydrogen bond interactions with Arg 120 having bond lengths (BL = 2.856 Å and BL = 2.835 Å) respectively. A decrease in antiplatelet activity of ASA was seen in the presence of tolmetin in the invitro experiments.

Figure 11a-f: Docking of NSAIDs which did not decrease the antiplatelet activity of ASA in the invitro experiments. Atom type colour code: Carbon=grey, chlorine=green, fluorine=skyblue, nitrogen=blue, oxygen=red, sulfur=yellow.

a. Acetaminophen:

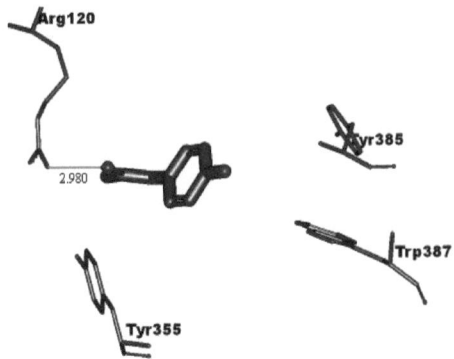

Acetaminophin forms only one hydrogen bond interactions with Arg 120 (BL = 2.980 Å). In the presence of acetaminophen, the in vitro experimental results did not show a decrease in antiplatelet activity of ASA.

b. Diclofenac:

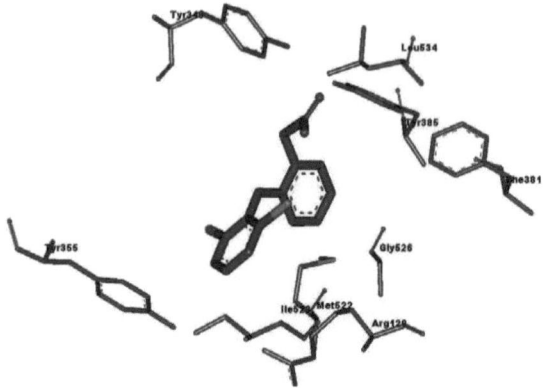

Diclofenac did not show any hydrogen bond interactions with Tyr 385, Ser 530, Arg 120 Tyr 355 and Trp 387. Diclofenac did not show a decrease in the antiplatelet activity of ASA in the in vitro experiments.

c. Flurbiprofen:

Flurbiprofen forms 3 hydrogen bond interactions, one with Tyr 355 (BL = 2.839 Å) and two with Arg 120 (BL = 2.638 Å and BL = 3.102 Å). In the presence of flurbiprofen ther was no decrease in antiplatelet activity of ASA in the in vitro experiments.

d. Indomethacin:

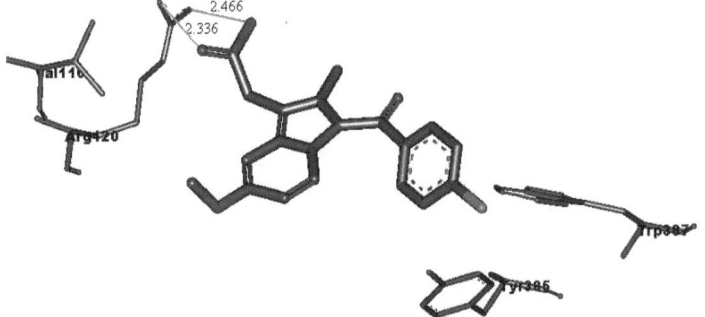

Indomethacin forms 2 hydrogen bond interactions with Arg 120 (BL = 2.466 Å and BL = 2.336 Å). The presence of indomethacin did not show a decrease in the antiplatelet activity of ASA in the in vitro experiments.

e. Ketoprofen:

Ketoprofen did not show any hydrogen bond interactions with Tyr 385, Ser 530, Arg 120 Tyr 355 and Trp 387. The presence of ketoprofen did not decrease antiplatelet activity of ASA in the in vitro experiments.

f. Ketorolac:

Ketorolac did not form any hydrogen bond interactions with Tyr 385, Ser 530, Arg 120 Tyr 355 and Trp 387. Ketorolac did not decrease antiplatelet activity of ASA in the in vitro experiments.

4. DISCUSSION

This thesis revealed several important results. These are the following. First, the majority of the studied NSAIDs, including celecoxib, fenoprofen, flufenamic acid, ibuprofen, mefenamic acid, nabumetone, naproxen, nimesulide, NS-398, oxaprozin, proyphenazone, phenazone, piroxicam, sulindac and tolmetin showed a decrease in the antiplatelet activity of ASA in the in vitro experiments with platelet rich plasma. Second, there was no decrease in antiplatelet activity of ASA in the presence of diclofenac, flurbiprofen, indomethacin, ketoprofen and ketorolac. Third, hydrogen bond interactions of the studied NSAIDs with amino acids within the COX-1 substrate channel (Ser 530, Tyr 385, Arg 120, Tyr 355, and Trp 387) may play a role in determining whether a drug will have an effect on the antiplatelet activity of ASA or not.

NSAID/ASA interactions have been long discussed. Thirty years ago, Livio and coworkers reported that indomethacin prevents the inhibitory effect of ASA using ram seminal COX-1 and rat platelets[36]. Subsequent studies also reported interactions with other NSAIDs. Studies by Catella-Lawson[27], Schuijit and coworkers[42] and Gladding[35] showed a decrease in antiplatelet activity of ASA in presence of NSAIDs in healthy subjects. However, the mechanism involved in this interaction is still not completely understood. The present thesis extends this previous work by studying a large number of NSAIDs and by examining possible molecular reasons for decrease in antiplatelet activity of ASA by NSAIDs.

The possible interactions which can cause a decrease in antiplatelet activity of ASA in presence of NSAIDs can be at following levels:

a) Impaired intestinal absorption of ASA

b) Impaired cell membrane transport

c) Pharmacodynamic interaction at the level of COX-1

d) Increased rate of inactivation

Since the interaction of NSAIDs and ASA was observed in vitro, an interaction at the level of NSAID absorption (a) and inactivation (d) is unlikely. Moreover, a previous study from our laboratory[34] demonstrated that the interaction between dipyrone (a nonselective COX inhibitor with analgesic but little anti-inflammatory activity) occurs not only in platelet rich plasma but also in a cell-free system using human platelet microsomal membranes. Moreover, dipyrone did not interfere in this study with a thromboxane synthase inhibitor. This suggests an interaction of dipyrone at the level of the COX-I enzyme rather than transport across platelet membranes. The present work confirms the interaction of dipyrone with ASA and shows that many other NSAIDs inferfere with ASA in a very similar manner. Hence, it is likely that the ASA/NSAID interaction occurs by a pharmacodynamic competition with ASA at the level of the platelet COX-I enzyme.

4.1 Discussion of the in vitro experimental results

The results show that many commonly administered NSAIDs attenuate or even prevent the antiplatelet action of ASA, as determined both by platelet function (aggregation) as well as biochemically (thromboxane formation) under well controlled experimental conditions.

The concentrations of the NSAIDs observed to interact with ASA are therapeutically relevant. For example, ibuprofen, naproxen and nimesulide achieve peak plasma concentrations (C_{max}) of 69, 47 and 15 µmol/L, respectively after administration of standard analgesic doses [79-81]. This is well within the range of NSAID concentrations applied in vitro in the present work. Celecoxib, fenoprofen, flufenamic acid mefanamic acid, metamizol, oxaprozin, piroxicam, phenazone, propyphenazone, sulindac, tolmetin and 6-MNA decreased the anti-platelet activity of ASA also at micromolar concentrations, which are generally achieved by routine therapeutic doses (see table 7).

The interaction of the NSAIDs with ASA occurred already at low micromolar or nanomolar concentrations, which did not (or minimally) inhibit platelet aggregation and thromboxane synthesis in the absence of ASA. The assumed interaction by NSAIDs is supported by a relatively low potency of ASA for inhibition of COX-1[66]. Although precise data of the studied NSAIDs for the inhibition kinetics of the platelet COX enzyme are not available, it is likely that these compounds effectively interfere with ASA at low concentrations. In contrast, arachidonic acid has a much higher COX-1 affinity[34] and is formed at high amounts upon platelet activation, so that low micromolar NSAID concentrations are not sufficient for platelet COX-1 inhibition.

The observed NSAID interactions with ASA were generally concentration-dependent, with the exception that the highest concentrations of some NSAIDs (ibuprofen, naproxen, nimesulide, oxaprozin) produced a decline of aggregation and TXB_2 formation, resulting in bell-shaped dose-response curves. This may be explained by the fact that lower concentrations of these NSAIDs predominantly prevented COX acetylation by ASA, while high concentrations moderately inhibit platelet COX-1 by themselves.

Table 7: Plasma concentrations (Cmax) obtained after commonly used therapeutic doses of the studied NSAIDs, as reported in the literature:

NSAID	Cmax (µmol/L)	References
Celecoxib	1.43	82
Dipyrone	50.7	83
Diclofenac	2.1	84
Fenoprofen	190	85
Flurbiprofen	40.5	79
Flufenamic acid	71.2	86
Ibuprofen	69.0	79
Indomethacin	11.9	87
Ketoprofen	10.2	88
Ketorolac	10.6	89
Mefenamic acid	15.0	90
Nabumetone (parent drug with first-pass metabolism to 6-MNA)	< 4.4	91
Naproxen	205.2	80
Nimesulide	15.2	81
Acetaminophin	141.1	92
Phenazone	70.7	93
Piroxicam	5.4	94
Propyphenazone	7.0	95
Oxaprozin	430	96
Sulindac sulfide	4.7	97
SC 560	0.54	98
Tolmetin	156	99
6-MNA (active metabolite of nabumetone)	192.5	91

The present study observed some interindividual variation from subject to subject, which likely reflect differences in plasma protein binding of the added NSAIDs, resulting in different free concentrations. Moreover, there may be interindividual differences in the sensitivity of platelets to stimulation by arachidonic acid and, possibly, genetic differences of the COX-1 enzyme. The limited number of subjects which were available did not allow to further examine the reason for the individual variability.

While several earlier studies have demonstrated that NSAIDs may prevent the antiplatelet effects of ASA, little is known about the comparative potential of NSAIDs to interfere with ASA. One exception is a recent study by Schuijt and coworkers, who administered repeated doses of low-dose ASA in combination either with ibuprofen or diclofenac to healthy subjects. These authors reported that ibuprofen alleviated ASA-induced inhibition of platelet thromboxane formation, while diclofenac did not[42]. It was hypothesized that diclofenac's relative COX-II selectivity may have allowed aspirin to interact with platelet COX-I, while ibuprofen due to its preferential COX-I selectivity may have prevented ASA to inhibit platelet COX-I. An additional study by Catella-Lawson and coworkers also reported that diclofenac, as well as acetaminophen, did not prevent platelet inhibition by ASA in healthy subjects[27]. They argued that this may reflect a shorter duration of action or lower potency of diclofenac compared with ibuprofen. Another study, comparing 6 NSAIDs given in conjunction with ASA to healthy subjects reported an attenuation of ASA's antiplatelet effect by ibuprofen, indomethacin, naproxen and tiaprofenic acid, but not by celecoxib and sulindac[35]. All these studies suggested that individual NSAIDs differentially interfere with ASA, but none could provide a definitve explanation of differences between individual compounds.

The in vitro design of our present study confirms this, clearly showing that among a comprehensive selection of NSAIDs (more than ever reported before), there are remarkable pharmacodynamic differences between different NSAIDs with respect to interaction with platelet inhibition by ASA. In contrast to many other conventional NSAIDs, diclofenac, indomethacin, flurbiprofen, ketoprofen, ketorolac and acetaminophin did not interfere with ASA at a broad range of concentrations below or higher than the clinically achieved plasma concentrations (see Table 7). Hence, the present results demonstrate that the interaction with ASA is *not* a class effect of all NSAIDs.

4.2 QSAR results discussion:

In addition to the described experimental results, a separate QSAR analysis has been performed which aimed to (i) cross validate the experimental results, (ii) determine the role of the IC_{50} or relative COX-1/COX-2 selectivity of the studied NSAIDs (both obtained from the literature[76]) for interference with ASA´s antiplatelet activity and (iii) to examine whether a combined effect of IC_{50} and COX-1/COX-2 selectivity may be related to the NSAIDs interference with the antiplatelet activity of ASA.

The QSAR model revealed the following points:

(i) There was a strong correlation between the NSAID concentration required for a 25% increase in aggregation and 25% increase in TXB_2 formation.

(ii) COX-I affinity (IC_{50}) or COX subtype selectivity (COX-1/COX-2 inhibition ratio) alone are not related to the NSAID interaction with ASA. Further, the QSAR analysis considered a resultant effect of both above mentioned factors in combination, as shown in table 5.

(iii) There seems to be a combined effect of the IC_{50} and COX-I/COX-II selectivity on NSAID/ASA interference. The NSAIDs with lower COX-I IC_{50} values than ASA and more selectivity towards COX-I over COX-II appear to be less likely to interfere with ASA, while those with a higher COX-I IC_{50} and lesser COX-I/COX-II selectivity more likely do interfere with ASA (see table 5).

4.3 Docking results discussion

In order to explain the interference by different NSAIDs in the anti-platelet action of ASA the following observations were of relevance: i) both ASA- and NSAID-binding sites lie within the narrow hydrophobic COX-I channel, ii) ASA acts by irreversibly acetylating a serine residue at position 530 and iii) all other NSAIDs, unlike ASA, bind reversibly within or at the entry of the hydrophobic channel.

The irreversible acetylation of COX-I by ASA involves an initial reversible, relatively weak binding within the hydrophobic channel[66]. Thus, those NSAIDs which bind at this site likely compete with ASA binding. This may result in the protection of platelet COX-I from permanent inactivation by ASA. The hydrophobic channel of COX-I has a length of 25 $Å$[20]. It originates at the membrane binding domain and extends into the core of the catalytic domain. The long hydrophobic channel has been divided into the 'lobby' and the substrate/inhibitor binding site, divided by the residues Arg-120, Glu-524, and Tyr-355, which form a constriction within the channel[20]. Most inhibitors bind at the COX active site near the constriction residues. Arg-120 is part of a hydrogen-bonding network with Glu-524 and Tyr-355, which stabilizes substrate/inhibitor interactions and closes off the upper part of the COX active site from the spacious opening at the base of the channel[20]. Disruption of this hydrogen-bonding network opens the constriction and enables substrate/inhibitor interactions[100]. In the existing X-ray crystal structures of COX-I with ASA (PDB ID: 1PTH[101]) the acetyl group of ASA is covalently bound to Ser-530. The product of the reaction, salicylic acid, is shown in the channel with its carboxylate making hydrogen bonds with Arg-120 and Tyr-355 at the constriction site (see Figure 12). The molecular basis of the interaction between ASA and NSAIDs, however, is not entirely clear. Thus, the present thesis addresses in a more detailed fashion the possibility of a structural explanation for the interference of the NSAIDs using in silico molecular modeling studies.

Figure 12: The co-crystallized structure of salicylic acid in COX-I (PDB ID: 1PTH) is involved in two hydrogen bonding intractions with Arg120 and Tyr355, respectively. Atom type colour code: Carbon=grey, chlorine=green, fluorine=skyblue, nitrogen=blue, oxygen=red, sulfur=yellow.

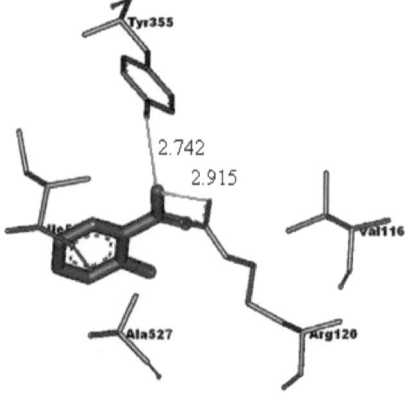

In order to carry out these docking studies the methodology has been validated by docking flurbiprofen in the hydrophobic channel and comparing the docked pose with the co-crystallized flurbiprofen (PDB ID: 1CQE) (Figure 9) where both were found similar in terms of pose and interaction. In view of ASA, Ser-530 is of particular importance because it is acetylated by ASA. Thus, those NSAIDs which show hydrogen bonding interaction with Ser-530 are most likely to interfere with the anti-platelet action of ASA. However, other amino acid residues within the hydrophobic channel may also play a role for accommodating the ligand in the hydrophobic channel.

Drugs showing interference in anti-platelet activity of ASA

Ibuprofen, mefenamic acid, nabumetone, naproxen, nimesulide, NS-398, oxaprozin, phenazone, piroxicam, sulindac, tolmentin, 6 MNA, diyprone (metamizol), propyphenazone and flufenamic acid were found to decrease the anti-platelet activity of aspirin in in-vitro experiments.

Among the 23 studied NSAIDs, the majority of compounds experimentally interfered with the inhibition of platelet aggregation and TXB_2 formation by ASA. However, the docking results demonstrated very different modes of binding within the hydrophobic channel.

The interfering compounds included all NSAIDs, which showed hydrogen bonding to Ser-530. This includes flufenamic acid, ibuprofen, MAA, mefenamic acid, nabumeton, nimesulide, NS-398, oxaprozin, phenazone, piroxicam, propyphenazon and sulindac sulfide. Since Ser-530 is the target of acetylation by ASA, the formation of hydrogen bonds at this site by NSAIDs most likely prevents the transfer of an acetyl group from ASA to this amino acid.

In addition to these NSAIDs, some others experimentally interfered with ASA without forming hydrogen bonding with Ser-530. It is long known that two other amino acids play a prominent role within the hydrophobic COX-I channel, as described above. These are Arg-120 and Tyr-355[20]. Among the NSAIDs interfering with ASA there are several which form hydrogen bonding with either Arg-120, Tyr-355 or both. These include celecoxib, MAA, fenoprofen, naproxen, sulindac, tolmetin, acetaminophen, flurbiprofen and indomethacin. The experimental results showed that many, but not all of them also interfere with platelet inhibiton by ASA. Thus, the docking results suggest that Arg-120 and Tyr-355 are of some importance for ASA interaction with COX-I, although this appears not as stringently connected with the experimental interaction with ASA as Ser-530. Therefore, some NSAIDs will be discussed separately as follows:

i) Celecoxib:

Celecoxib docking showed one hydrogen bond interaction with Tyr-355, one with Ile-517 and one with Phe-518. Tyr-355 is present in the active site and hence interaction of celecoxib with this residue likely results in decrease in anti-platelet activity of ASA. The other two hydrogen bond interactions may further stabilize the celecoxib docking. This docking conformation is consistent with a previous study by Rimon and coworkers derived from crystallography[37]. It may be of importance for COX-I inhibition by ASA, as demonstrated by the experimental data obtained in this study and previous results reported by others (eg: Rimon et al.[37]).

ii) Naproxen:

Naproxen showed one hydrogen bond interaction with Tyr 355 and one with Arg 120. Both Tyr 355 and Arg 120 are present in the active channel in COX-1 protein. Thus, naproxen may hinder the approach of ASA within the active channel and decreases the anti-platelet activity of ASA.

iii) Sulindac sulfide:

Sulindac docking showed one hydrogen bond interaction with Arg 120 and one with Tyr 355 and, in this respect, was similar with naproxen. Hence, these hydrogen bond interactions may hinder the approach of ASA in the active channel of COX-1 protein and decrease the antiplatelet activity of ASA.

iv) Tolmetin:

Tolmetin forms 2 hydrogen bond interactions with Arg 120. This may decrease the ability of aspirin to enter the active channel in COX-1, since Arg-120 is the site of initial reversible binding of ASA to COX-1[102] and hence may decrease the anti-platelet effect of ASA as shown experimentally.

Drugs not showing any decrease in anti-platelet activity of ASA:

Diclofenac, flurbiprofen, indomethacin, ketorolac and ketoprofen did not decrease the antiplatelet activity of ASA in the in vitro experiments. Among these diclofenac, ketoprofen and ketorolac docking did not reveal any hydrogen bond interactions with Arg-120, Ser-530, Tyr-385, Tyr-355 and Trp-387. Hence, they are likely to not hinder the binding of ASA at its catalytic site within the active channel in the COX-I protein.

Acetaminophen docking showed only one hydrogen bond interaction with Arg 120 within the active channel of COX-1 protein. A single hydrogen bond interaction with Arg 120 is probably not sufficient to hinder the approach of aspirin in the active channel of COX protein. This may be the reason for no effect of acetaminophen on the antiplatelet activity of ASA. Indomethacin and tolmetin both showed in docking two hydrogen bond interactions with Arg-120, but still did not decrease the antiplatelet activity of ASA. Similarly, flurbiprofen showed two hydrogen bond interaction with Arg-120 and one with Tyr-355 but it also didn't show interference with ASA's antiplatet activity.

The discussion of the interactive effect of tolmetin and absence of interactive effect of indomethacin requires consideration of bond-lengths. Indomethacin forms 2 hydrogen bonds (bond length = 2.336; 2.466 Å), thereby being more close to Arg-120 and hence more in the periphery of entrance of hydrophobic channel. In contrast, tolmetin forms 2 hydrogen bonds (bond length =2.856;2.835 Å) and hence is more centrally located in the hydrophobic channel. This may lead to more hindrance in the entrance of ASA into the active channel and potentially for this reason tolmetin interferes with the antiplatelet effect of ASA.

However, it is difficult to explain the reason behind no interference by flurbiprofen, which also shows two interactions with Arg-120 and one with Tyr-355. The phenyl group in flurbiprofen might have less steric hindrance in the passage of ASA within the active channel of COX and so the antiplatelet activity of ASA may remain unaffected.

4.4 Discussion of clinical implications

The problem of the NSAIDs/ASA interaction addressed in this thesis is of therapeutic importance because no routine monitoring of anti-platelet action of ASA has been established so far. Thus, individual patients affected by this interaction will probably not be identified. Routine monitoring of platelet function is even not recommended by the current guidelines for treatment of coronary artery disease.

The cessation of antiplatelet therapy with ASA may substantially increase atherothombotic events and impair clinical outcome in patients with cardiovascular disease[31,38-40]. A meta analysis of 6 trials studied the effect of stopping ASA on the rate of atherothrombosis[41]. In patients with stable coronary artery disease (3 trials) and patients after coronary artery surgery (2 trials), thrombotic events were about 2-fold increased. This was statistically significant in each of the trials. Stopping ASA in patients with coronary stents increased the risk of atherothrombosis more than 30-fold, reflecting that stent implantation imposes a particularly high risk of coronary thrombosis which underlines the particular importance of effective antiplatelet therapy in this patient subgroup.

There is evidence that both COX-I and COX-II inhibitors are associated with an increase in cardiovascular thrombosis and cerebral strokes. A common explanation is the hypothesis that NSAIDs may inhibit prostaglandin synthesis in the vascular wall. The major prostaglandin species formed in the vascular wall is prostacyclin (mostly COX-2 -dependent). PGI_2 has a potent antiplatelet effect, is vasodilatory and has antiinflammatoy properties. Hence, the common explanation of the increase of arterial thrombotic events associated with NSAIDs is the (unintended) inhibition of vascular prostacyclin formation[103]. This is plausible but there may also be other contributing factors, such as the interaction of NSAIDs with ASA.

Patients with pre-existing cardiovascular disease are likely to receive co-medication of NSAIDs with low dose ASA. Therefore, the NSAIDs may also have prevented ASA's antiplatelet effect. This explanation is supported by the Scottish Tayside trial, which studied cardiovascular mortality in more than 7000 patients with cardiovascular disease receiving low-dose ASA. This trial observed a significant increase of mortality in the subgroup receiving co-treatment with ibuprofen[104]. In line with the conclusion from the present thesis, diclofenac did not have any adverse influence on mortality. Accordingly, the TARGET trial, which examined cardiovascular outcome of patients receiving lumiracoxib, showed that ASA users on ibuprofen had more major cardiovascular events and developed more frequently congestive heart failure than ASA users not receiving ibuprofen[105]. Therefore, there is some support from clinical trials that some but possibly not all NSAIDs interfere with cardiovascular protection by ASA. A clinical trial which adresses this interaction in a prospective design, however, has not yet been performed.

4.5 Criticism of Methodology

The experimental results of this study were obtained by incubation of platelet rich plasma with the studied compounds in vitro with subsequent platelet activation by one well-defined stimulus (arachidonic acid). This certainly differs from the situation in vivo, where drugs are present for longer times with continuously changing plasma concentrations according to drug metabolism and elimination. Platelets are likely activated in biological systems by several stimuli other than arachidonic acid, such as thrombin, adenosine diphosphate (ADP), collagen and others. Therefore, clinical trials are required to examine whether NSAID/ASA interactions occur in clinical settings and whether these may have impact on clinical outcome. It should be mentioned, however, that a number of studies in healthy subjects as well as patients with vascular disease indeed did suggest a clincal importance of this interaction.

Another possible limitation is the docking analysis used in the present work, which focuses on the molecular interaction between the NSAIDs and their potential interactions with amino acids in the hydrophobic channel of COX-I but does not consider more complex mechanisms, such as potential secondary changes in protein conformation and interaction of the two subunits of the COX enzyme.

For example, it was demonstrated that some reversible competitive NSAIDs (e.g., ibuprofen) bind to both COX monomers for enzyme inhibition[106], thereby likely competing with ASA. However, other NSAIDs appear to bind only to one COX monomer, causing a structural change of the interface between the monomers. This may be followed by a secondary change of the substrate binding site, resulting in an inhibition of the partner monomer[107]. Recent work by Rimon an coworkers, who studied binding of celecoxib to COX isoforms by crystallography, suggested a change in the crosstalk between the two subunits[37].

While celecoxib also potently interfered with ASA in our in vitro experiments and the present docking analysis suggests that celecoxib forms hydrogen bonds to Tyr355, His513 and Ile517, a secondary effect on COX-subuunit crosstalk could not be addressed in our study. It should be noted, however, that most of the data reporting crosstalk between COX subunits have been generated with the COX-II isoenzyme, which may or may not be relevant for COX-I, the isoform largely expressed in platelets. Thus, it is currently not possible to determine whether spatial hindrance by NSAIDs due to formation of hydrogen bonds or a regulation of ligand affinity by inter-subunit crosstalk are the true mechanism of NSAID/ASA interaction.

In the statistical analysis of QSAR, it may be criticised that fenoprofen and oxaprozin were outlier which did not fit into the QSAR conclusions (see graph 3 and graph 5). This may suggest that these two NSAIDs act through an incompletely understood molecular mechanisms which is not covered by the present QSAR analysis (such as secondary effects on subunit crosstalk).

5. CONCLUSION

The present study shows that numerous NSAIDs, which are commonly used for analgesic, antiinflammatory and antipyretic indications, show a remarkable in vitro drug/drug interaction with ASA. This results in an attenuation or prevention of the antiplatelet effects of ASA, including the prevention of arachidonic induced platelet aggregation and inhibition of platelet TXB_2 formation. This is observed at NSAID concentrations which are well achieved during routine analgesic therapy. Hence, the observed in vitro interactions are likely of clinical relevance.

Interestingly, the in-vitro experiments also showed that some NSAIDs, including acetaminophen, diclofenac, fluribiprofen, indomethacin, ketoprofen and ketorolac, do *not* decrease the anti-platelet activity of ASA. These NSAIDs may be preferred in patients who take low dose of aspirin for secondary prevention of cerebral stroke or myocardial infarction, at least if given continuously over several days or longer.

Docking studies helped to provide some insight into the molecular mechanisms involved in NSAID/ASA interaction. From this part of the study it can be concluded that amino acids (Tyr 385, Ser 530, Arg 120, Tyr 355, Trp 387) present within the active channel of the COX-I protein likely play a vital role in determining whether a particular drug would decrease the anti-platelet activity of ASA or not. This and the QSAR results may be useful for designing other NSAIDs which would not decrease the anti-platelet activity of ASA. Further research should analyze the time-dependent and time-independent kinetics of each NSAID and its effect on the COX-I protein free energy, which might control the cross talk mechanism between the monomers of COX-I protein. There is also a chance that this thesis may be helpful for physicians to choose safer NSAIDs for patients taking ASA for prevention of myocardial infarction and cerebral ischemia.

6. REFERENCES

1. Campbell CL, Smyth S, Montalescot G, Steinhubl SR (2007) Aspirin dose for the prevention of cardiovascular disease: a systematic review. JAMA 297: 2018-2024.
2. Flossmann E, Rothwell PM (2007) Effect of aspirin on long-term risk of colorectal cancer: consistent evidence from randomised and observational studies. Lancet 369:1603-1603.
3. Cascorbi I (2012) Drug interactions--principles, examples and clinical consequences. Dtsch Ärztebl Int 109:546-555.
4. Cheng JW (2006) Use of non-aspirin nonsteroidal antiinflammatory drugs and the risk of cardiovascular events. Ann Pharmacother 40:1785-1796.
5. Schrör K (2009) Acetylsalicylic acid. Wiley, Weinheim, pp. 5-6.
6. Bachoffner P (1997) Two pharmacists in the beginning of Aspirin: Charles Gerhardt and Felix Hoffmann. Rev Hist Pharm 45:411-414.
7. Norn S, Permin H, Kruse PR, Kruse E (2009) From willow bark to acetylsalicylic acid. Dan Medicinhist Arbog 37:79-98.
8. Craven LL (1950) Acetylsalicylic acid, possible preventive of coronary thrombosis. Ann West Med Surg 4:95.
9. Gibson PC (1949) Aspirin in the treatment of vascular diseases. Lancet 2:1172-1174.
10. Craven LL (1956) Prevention of coronary and cerebral thrombosis. Miss Valley Med J 78:213-215.
11. Ridker PM, Cook NR, Lee IM, Gordon D, Gaziano JM, Manson JE, Hennekens CH, Buring JE (2005) A randomized trial of low-dose aspirin in the primary prevention of cardiovascular disease in women. N Engl J Med 352:1293-1304.
12. Antithrombotic Trialists' Collaboration (2002) Collaborative meta-analysis of randomised trials of antiplatelet therapy for prevention of death, myocardial infarction, and stroke in high risk patients. BMJ 324:71-86.
13. Vane JR, Botting RM (2003) The mechanism of action of aspirin. Thromb Res 110:255-258.
14. Jerie P (2006) Milestones of cardiovascular pharmacotherapy: salicylates and aspirin. Cas Lek Cesk 145:901-904.

15. Karow T, Lang-roth R (2007) Allgemeine und Spezielle Pharmakologie und Toxikologie., Lang, Pulheim, pp. 532-536
16. Tosco P, Lazzarato L (2009) Mechanistic insights into cyclooxygenase irreversible inactivation by aspirin. ChemMedChem 4: 939-945
17. Censarek P, Freidel K, Udelhoven M, Ku SJ, Hohlfeld T, Meyer-Kirchrath J, Schrör K, Weber AA (2004) Cyclooxygenase COX-2a, a novel COX-2 mRNA variant, in platelets from patients after coronary artery bypass grafting. Thromb Haemost 92:925-928.
18. Mitchell JA, Akarasereenont P, Thiemermann C, Flower RJ, Vane JR (1993) Selectivity of nonsteroidal antiinflammatory drugs as inhibitors of constitutive and inducible cyclooxygenase. Proc Natl Acad Sci 90:11693-11697.
19. Fiorucci S, Distrutti E, de Lima OM, Romano M, Mencarelli A, Barbanti M, Palazzini E, Morelli A, Wallace JL (2003) Relative contribution of acetylated cyclo-oxygenase (COX)-2 and 5-lipooxygenase (LOX) in regulating gastricmucosal integrity and adaptation to aspirin.FASEB J 9:1171-1173.
20. Picot D, Loll PJ, Garavito RM (1994) The X-ray crystal structure of the membrane protein prostaglandin H2 synthase-1. Nature 367:243-249.
21. Meade EA, Smith WL, DeWitt DL (1993) Differential inhibition of prostaglandin endoperoxide synthase (cyclooxygenase) isozymes by aspirin and other non-steroidal anti-inflammatory drugs. J Biol Chem 268:6610-6614.
22. McCarty MF, Block KI (2006) Preadministration of high-dose salicylates, suppressors of NF-kappaB activation, may increase the chemosensitivity of many cancers: an example of proapoptotic signal modulation therapy. Integr Cancer Ther 3:252-268.
23. Sørensen HT, Mellemkjaer L, Blot WJ, Nielsen GL, Steffensen FH, McLaughlin JK, Olsen JH (2000) Risk of upper gastrointestinal bleeding associated with use of low-dose aspirin. Am J Gastroenterol 9:2218-2224.
24. Szczeklik A, Stevenson DD (2003) Aspirin-induced asthma: advances in pathogenesis, diagnosis, and management. J Allergy Clin Immunol 111:913-921.

25. Schrör K (2007) Aspirin and Reye Syndrome: A Review of the Evidence. Pediatric Drugs 9:195-204.
26. Schrör K (2009) Acetylsalicylic acid. Wiley, Weinheim, pp. 41-42.
27. Catella-Lawson F, Reilly MP, Kapoor SC, Cucchiara AJ, DeMarco S, Tournier B, Vyas SN, FitzGerald GA (2001) Cyclooxygenase inhibitors and the antiplatelet effects of aspirin. N Engl J Med 345:1809-1817.
28. Yeung J, Holinstat M (2012) Newer agents in antiplatelet therapy: a review. J Blood Med 3:33-42.
29. Dalen JE (2006) Aspirin to prevent heart attack and stroke: what's the right dose? Am J Med 119:198-202.
30. Symmons DP, Gabriel SE (2011) Epidemiology of CVD in rheumatic disease, with a focus on RA and SLE. Nat Rev Rheumatol 7:399-408.
31. Gengo FM, Rubin L, Robson M, Rainka M, Gengo MF, Mager DE, Bates V (2008) Effects of ibuprofen on the magnitude and duration of aspirin's inhibition of platelet aggregation: clinical consequences in stroke prophylaxis. J Clin Pharmacol 48 :117-122.
32. Capone ML, Sciulli MG, Tacconelli S, Grana M, Ricciotti E, Renda G, Di Gregorio P, Merciaro G, Patrignani P (2005) Pharmacodynamic interaction of naproxen with low-dose aspirin in healthy subjects. JACC 45:1295-1301.
33. Anzellotti P, Capone ML, Jeyam A, Tacconelli S, Bruno A, Tontodonati P, Di Francesco L, Grossi L, Renda G, Merciaro G, Di Gregorio P, Price TS, Garcia Rodriguez LA, Patrignani P (2011) Low-dose naproxen interferes with the antiplatelet effects of aspirin in healthy subjects: recommendations to minimize the functional consequences. Arthritis Rheum 63:850-859.
34. Hohlfeld T, Zimmermann N, Weber AA, Jessen G, Weber H, Schrör K, Höltje HD, Ebel R (2008) Pyrazolinone analgesics prevent the antiplatelet effect of aspirin and preserve human platelet thromboxane synthesis. J Thromb Haemost 6:166-173.
35. Gladding PA, Webster MW, Farrell HB, Zeng IS, Park R, Ruijne N (2008) The antiplatelet effect of six non-steroidal anti-inflammatory drugs and their pharmacodynamic interaction with aspirin in healthy volunteers. Am J Cardiol 101:1060-1063.

36. Livio M, Del Maschio A, Cerletti C, de Gaetano G (1982) Indomethacin prevents the long-lasting inhibitory effect of aspirin on human platelet cyclo-oxygenase activity. Prostaglandins 23:787-796.
37. Rimon G, Sidhu RS, Lauver DA, Lee JY, Sharma NP, Yuan C, Frieler RA, Trievel RC, Lucchesi BR, Smith WL (2010) Coxibs interfere with the action of aspirin by binding tightly to one monomer of cyclooxygenase-1. Proc Natl Acad Sci 107:28-33.
38. Grotemeyer KH, Scharafinski HW, Husstedt IW (1993) Two-year follow-up of aspirin responder and aspirin non responder. A pilot-study including 180 post-stroke patients. Thromb Res 71:397-403.
39. Mueller MR, Salat A, Stangl P, Murabito M, Pulaki S, Boehm D, Koppensteiner R, Ergun E, Mittlboeck M, Schreiner W, Losert U, Wolner E (1997) Variable platelet response to low-dose ASA and the risk of limb deterioration in patients submitted to peripheral arterial angioplasty. Thromb Haemost 78:1003-1007.
40. Gaede P, Vedel P, Larsen N, Jensen GV, Parving HH, Pedersen O (2003) Multifactorial Intervention and Cardiovascular Disease in Patients with Type 2 Diabetes. N Engl J Med 348:383-393.
41. Biondi-Zoccai GG, Lotrionte M, Agostoni P, Abbate A, Fusaro M, Burzotta F, Testa L, Sheiban I, Sangiorgi G (2006) A systematic review and meta-analysis on the hazards of discontinuing or not adhering to aspirin among 50,279 patients at risk for coronary artery disease. Eur Heart J 27:2667-2674.
42. Schuijt MP, Huntjens-Fleuren HW, de Metz M, Vollaard EJ (2009) The interaction of ibuprofen and diclofenac with aspirin in healthy volunteers. Br J Pharmacol 157:931-934.
43. Renda G, Tacconelli S, Capone ML, Sacchetta D, Santarelli F, Sciulli MG, Zimarino M, Grana M, D'Amelio E, Zurro M, Price TS, Patrono C, De Caterina R, Patrignani P (2006) Celecoxib, ibuprofen, and the antiplatelet effect of aspirin in patients with osteoarthritis and ischemic heart disease. Clin Pharmacol Ther 80:264-274.
44. Biagi GL, Guerra MC, Barbaro AM, Gamba MF (1970) Influence of lipophilic character on the antibacterial activity of cephalosporins and penicillins. J Med Chem 13:511-516.

45. Snyder JP (1991) Drug Design, Searle Research & Development, Skokie, Illinois. Med Res Rev 11:641-662.
46. Hollenberg MD (1990) Receptor triggering and receptor regulation: structure-activity relationships from the receptor's point of view. J Med Chem 33:1275-1281.
47. A. J. Hopfinger(1985) Computer-assisted drug design. J. Med. Chem 28. 1133–1139.
48. Kuntz ID, Blaney JM, Oatley SJ, Langridge R, Ferrin TE (1982) A geometric approach to macromolecule-ligand interactions. J Mol Biol 161:269-288.
49. Morris GM, Goodsell DS, Huey R, Olson AJ (1996) Distributed automated docking of flexible ligands to proteins: parallel applications of AutoDock 2.4. J Comput Aided Mol Des 10:293-304.
50. Abagyan, R.A., Totrov, M.M., Kuznetsov, D.A (1994) ICM: a new method for structure modeling and design: Applications to docking and structure prediction from the distorted native conformation. J. Comp. Chem 15:488–506.
51. Jones G, Willett P, Glen RC, Leach AR, Taylor R (1997) Development and validation of a genetic algorithm for flexible docking. J Mol Biol 267:727-748.
52. Rarey M, Kramer B, Lengauer T, Klebe G (1996) A fast flexible docking method using an incremental construction algorithm. J Mol Biol 261:470-489.
53. Gabb HA, Jackson RM, Sternberg MJ (1997) Modelling protein docking using shape complementarity, electrostatics and biochemical information. J Mol Biol 272:106-120.
54. Burkhard P, Taylor P, Walkinshaw MD (1998) An example of a protein ligand found by database mining: description of the docking method and its verification by a 2.3 A X-ray structure of a thrombin-ligand complex. J Mol Biol 277:449-466.
55. Crum-Brown A, Fraser TR (1868) On the connection between chemical constitution and physiological action. Trans Roy Soc Edinburgh 25:151–203.
56. Meyer, H (1899) Zur theorie der alkoholnarkose. Arch. Exp. Pathol. Pharmakol. 42:109-118.
57. Overton E (1901) Studien über die Narkose. Gustav Fischer Verlag, Jena.

58. Ferguson, J (1939) The use of chemical potentials as indices of toxicity. Proc. R Soc 127:387-404.
59. Hammett LP (1940) Physical Organic Chemistry. McGraw Hill, New York.
60. Draper NR, Smith H (1966) Applied regression analysis. Wiley, New York.
61. Miller AJ (1990) Subset Selection in Regression, Chapman and Hall, London.
62. Pearlman RS, Yalkowsky SH, Sinkula AA, Valvani YC (1980) Physical Chemical Properties of Drugs. Dekker, New York.
63. Weiner PK, Kollman PA (1981) AMBER: Assisted Model Building with Energy Refinement. A General Program for Modeling Molecules and Their Interactions. J Comp Chem 2:287-303.
64. Martin YC, Bustard TM, Lynn KR (1973) Relationship between physical properties and antimalarial activities of 1,4-naphthoquinones. J Med Chem 10:1089-1093.
65. Goltsov A, Maryashkin A, Swat M, Kosinsky Y, Humphery-Smith I, Demin O, Goryanin I, Lebedeva G (2009) Kinetic modelling of NSAID action on COX-1: focus on in vitro/in vivo aspects and drug combinations. Eur J Pharm Sci 36:122-136.
66. Marc Ouellet, Denis Riendeau, M. David Percival (2001) A high level of cyclooxygenase-2 inhibitor selectivity is associated with a reduced interference of platelet cyclooxygenase-1 inactivation by aspirin. Proc Natl Acad Sci 98:14583–14588.
67. Thomsen R, Christensen MH (2006) MolDock: a new technique for high accuracy molecular docking. J Med Chem 49:3315–3321.
68. Storn R, Price K (1995) Differential evolution-A Simple and Efficient Adaptive Scheme for Global Optimization over continuous spaces. International Computer Science Institute press, Berkley.
69. Gehlhaar DK, Verkhivker G, Rejto PA, Fogel DB, Fogel LJ, Freer ST (1995) Proceedings of the Fourth Annual Conference on Evolutionary Programming. MIT Press, Cambridge, pp 615-627.
70. Gehlhaar DK, Verkhivker GM, Rejto PA, Sherman CJ, Fogel DB, Fogel LJ, Freer ST (1995) Molecular recognition of the inhibitor AG-1343 by HIV-1 protease: conformationally flexible docking by evolutionary programming. Chem Biol 2:317–324.

71. Gehlhaar DK, Bouzida D, Rejto PA (1998) Proceedings of the seventh international conference on evolutionary programming. Springer, Berlin, pp. 449-461.
72. Loll PJ, Picot D, Ekabo O, Garavito RM (1996) Synthesis and use of iodinated nonsteroidal antiinflammatory drug analogs as crystallographic probes of the prostaglandin H2 synthase cyclooxygenase active site. Biochemistry 35:7330-7340.
73. http://www.rcsb.org/pdb/explore/explore.do?structureId=1PGG. Access date: January 16, 2013
74. http://accelrys.com/products/discovery-studio/ Access date: January 16, 2013
75. http://www.rcsb.org/pdb/explore/explore.do?structureId=1CQE Access date: January 16, 2013
76. Cryer B, Feldman M (1998) Cyclooxygenase-1 and cyclooxygenase-2 selectivity of widely used nonsteroidal anti-inflammatory drugs. Am J Med 104:413-421.
77. http://www.systat.com/ Access date: January 16, 2013
78. Schmitt KC, Reith ME (2011) The atypical stimulant and nootropic modafinil interacts with the dopamine transporter in a different manner than classical cocaine-like inhibitors. PLoS One 6:e25790
79. Pargal A, Kelkar MG, Nayak PJ (1996) The effect of food on the bioavailability of ibuprofen and flurbiprofen from sustained release formulations. Biopharm Drug Dispos 6:511-519.
80. Zhou D, Zhang Q, Lu W, Xia Q, Wei S (1998) Single- and multiple-dose pharmacokinetic comparison of a sustained-release tablet and conventional tablets of naproxen in healthy volunteers. J Clin Pharmacol 7:625-629.
81. Bernareggi A (1998) Clinical pharmacokinetics of nimesulide. Clin Pharmacokinet 35:247-274.
82. Jayasagar G, Krishna Kumar M, Chandrasekhar K, Madhusudan Rao Y (2003) Influence of rifampicin pretreatment on the pharmacokinetics of celecoxib in healthy male volunteers. Drug Metabol Drug Interact 19:287-295.
83. Suarez-Kurtz G, Ribeiro FM, Estrela RC, Vicente FL, Struchiner CJ (2001) Limited-sampling strategy models for estimating the pharmacokinetic

parameters of 4-methylaminoantipyrine, an active metabolite of dipyrone. Braz J Med Biol Res 34:1475-1485.

84. Raz I, Hussein Z, Samara E, Ben-David J (1988) Comparative pharmacokinetic analysis of a novel sustained-release dosage form of diclofenac sodium in healthy subjects. Int J Clin Pharmacol Ther Toxicol 26: 246-248.

85. Barissa GR, Poggi JC, Donadi EA, Dos Reis ML, Lanchote VL (2004) Influence of rheumatoid arthritis in the enantioselective disposition of fenoprofen. Chirality 16:602-608.

86. Lentjes EG, van Ginneken CA (1987) Pharmacokinetics of flufenamic acid in man. Int J Clin Pharmacol Ther Toxicol 25:185-187.

87. Bruguerolle B, Barbeau G, Bélanger PM, Labrecque G (1986) Pharmacokinetics of a sustained-release product of indomethacin in the elderly. Gerontology 32:277-285.

88. Rolf C, Engström B, Beauchard C, Jacobs LD, Le Liboux A (1999) Intra-articular absorption and distribution of ketoprofen after topical plaster application and oral intake in 100 patients undergoing knee arthroscopy. Rheumatology 38:564-567.

89. Jung D, Mroszczak EJ, Wu A, Ling TL, Sevelius H, Bynum L (1989) Pharmacokinetics of ketorolac and p-hydroxyketorolac following oral and intramuscular administration of ketorolac tromethamine. Pharm Res 6:62-65.

90. Hamaguchi T, Shinkuma D, Yamanaka Y, Mizuno N (1986) Bioavailability of mefenamic acid: influence of food and water intake. J Pharm Sci 75:891-893.

91. Kendall MJ, Chellingsworth MC, Jubb R, Thawley AR, Undre NA, Kill DC (1989) A pharmacokinetic study of the active metabolite of nabumetone in young healthy subjects and older arthritis patients. Eur J Clin Pharmacol 36:299-305.

92. Critchley JA, Critchley LA, Anderson PJ, Tomlinson B (2005)Differences in the single-oral-dose pharmacokinetics and urinary excretion of paracetamol and its conjugates between Hong Kong Chinese and Caucasian subjects. J Clin Pharm Ther 30:179-184.

93. Greenblatt DJ, Divoll MK, Harmatz JS, Shader RI (1988) Antipyrine absorption and disposition in the elderly. Pharmacology 36:125-133.

94. Wang D, Miller R, Zheng J, Hu C (2000) Comparative population pharmacokinetic-pharmacodynamic analysis for piroxicam-beta-cyclodextrin and piroxicam. J Clin Pharmacol 40:1257-1266.
95. Volz M, Kellner HM (1980) Kinetics and metabolism of pyrazolones (propyphenazone, aminopyrine and dipyrone). Br J Clin Pharmacol 10:299-308.
96. Chiang ST, Knowles JA, Hubsher JA, Ruelius HW, Walker BR (1984) Effects of food on oxaprozin bioavailability. J Clin Pharmacol 24:381-385.
97. Swanson BN, Boppana VK, Vlasses PH, Holmes GI, Monsell K, Ferguson RK (1982) Sulindac disposition when given once and twice daily. Clin Pharmacol Ther 32:397-403.
98. Teng XW, Davies NM (2004) High-performance liquid chromatographic analysis of a selective cyclooxygenase-1 inhibitor SC-560 in rat serum: application to pharmacokinetic studies. J Pharm Biomed Anal 35:1143-1147.
99. http://doublecheckmd.com/DrugDetail.do?dname=Tolectin+DS&sid=4495& view=pk Access date: January 16, 2013
100. Luong C, Miller A, Barnett J, Chow J, Ramesha C, Browner MF (1996) Flexibility of the NSAID binding site in the structure of human cyclooxygenase-2. Nat Struct Biol 3:927-933.
101. PDB ID: 1PTH
102. Loll PJ, Picot D, Garavito RM (1995) The structural basis of aspirin activity inferred from the crystal structure of inactivated prostaglandin H2 synthase. Nat Struct Biol 2:637-643.
103. Grosser T, Fries S, FitzGerald GA (2006) Biological basis for the cardiovascular consequences of COX-2 inhibition: therapeutic challenges and opportunities. J Clin Invest 116:4-15.
104. MacDonald TM, Wei L (2003) Effect of ibuprofen on cardioprotective effect of aspirin. Lancet 361:573-574.
105. Farkouh ME, Greenberg JD, Jeger RV, Ramanathan K, Verheugt FW, Chesebro JH, Kirshner H, Hochman JS, Lay CL, Ruland S, Mellein B, Matchaba PT, Fuster V, Abramson SB (2007) Cardiovascular outcomes in high risk patients with osteoarthritis treated with ibuprofen, naproxen or lumiracoxib. Ann Rheum Dis 66:764-770.

106. Sharma NP, Dong L, Yuan C, Noon KR, Smith WL (2010) Asymmetric acetylation of the cyclooxygenase-2 homodimer by aspirin and its effects on the oxygenation of arachidonic, eicosapentaenoic, and docosahexaenoic acids. Mol Pharmacol 77:979-986.
107. Smith WL, Urade Y, Jakobsson PJ (2011) Enzymes of the cyclooxygenase pathways of prostanoid biosynthesis. Chem Rev 111:5821-5865.
108. Hohlfeld T, Saxena A, Schrör K (2012) High on treatment platelet reactivity against aspirin by non-steroidal anti-inflammatory drugs - pharmacological mechanisms and clinical relevance. Thromb Haemost. 13;109.

7. CURRICULUM VITAE

Personal Information

Surname	:	Saxena
First name	:	Aaruni
Date of birth	:	03.08.1981
Place of birth	:	Lucknow, Indien
Citizenship	:	Indien
Address	:	Stendaler strasse 20, 40599, Düsseldorf
Tel	:	0049-15118115165
Email	:	aaruni85@rediffmail.com

School Education

1985- 1997	:	The Lucknow Public Collegiate(ISCE)
1997- 1999	:	City Montessori School ,Gomti Nagar, Lucknow (ISC)

University Education

2000 - 2002	:	University of Medicine and Pharmacy ,Timisoara
2003 - 2007	:	University of Rostock (Humanmedizin)
2007 - 2008	:	Practical internship (PJ) in Universität Rostock
01/2011	:	2 ärztliche Prüfung
2008 - 2013	:	Henrich Heine Universität Düsseldorf (Research) Institute of Pharmacology and Clinical Pharmacology

Practicum

1999-2000	:	Krishna Public Collegiate , Kashipur, Indien

Clinical Training

02/ 2007 -05/ 2007	:	All India Institute of Medical Sciences (AIIMS), Department of Internal medicine, Newdelhi, Indien
06/ 2007-07/2007	:	All India Institute of Medical Sciences (AIIMS), Department of Surgery, Newdelhi, Indien
08/ 2007-09/2007	:	University of Rostock, department of Surgery
10/2008 - 01/2008	:	University of Rostock, Orthopaedics department.

Residency

05/2012 -08/2012	:	St. Vinzenz Krankenhaus, Düsseldorf.
Seit 01/2013	:	Katharine Hospital, Willich.

Foreign language

German	:	Zentral Mittelstufeprüfung „ZMP"
English	:	IELTS
French	:	A1 level

Hobbys

Sport	:	Football, Cricket

8. ACKNOWLEDGEMENT

I would like to convey my thanks to Prof. Dr .med. Thomas hohlfeld, Institute of pharmacology and clinical pharmacology, University of Duesseldorf, to provide me opportunity to do work in the field of aspirin/ NSAIDs interaction under his guidance.

I would like to thank our ex-director Prof. Dr.med. Karsten Schrör for his constant support and encouragement.

My thanks to our present director Prof. Dr. Jens W. Fischer, who supported our research work and also provided platform to present our research work in many international conferences and scientific meet.

I would also like to extend my thanks to Prof. Dr. Holger Gohlke, Institute of pharmaceutical and medicinal chemistry, University of Duesseldorf and to Dr. Anil Kumar Saxena, Scientist F, Central drug research institute, India for their expert advices and guidance in field of molecular modeling and QSAR (Quantitative structural analysis relationship).

At last but not the least, I would like to thank Ms. Kirsten Bartkowski, CTA, Institute of pharmacology and clinical pharmacology, University of Duesseldorf, for experimental studies and her constant support throughout my research work.

My sincere gratitude is towards all my seniors and colleagues in the Institute of pharmacology and clinical pharmacology for standing with me throughout my research thesis work and stay in the institute.

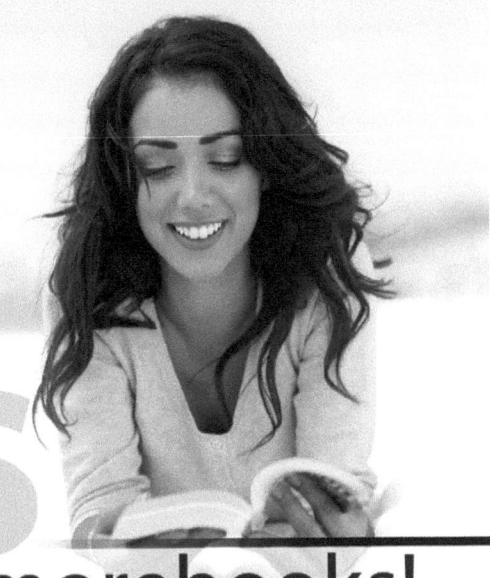

I want morebooks!

Buy your books fast and straightforward online - at one of the world's fastest growing online book stores! Environmentally sound due to Print-on-Demand technologies.

Buy your books online at

www.get-morebooks.com

Kaufen Sie Ihre Bücher schnell und unkompliziert online – auf einer der am schnellsten wachsenden Buchhandelsplattformen weltweit! Dank Print-On-Demand umwelt- und ressourcenschonend produziert.

Bücher schneller online kaufen

www.morebooks.de

OmniScriptum Marketing DEU GmbH
Heinrich-Böcking-Str. 6 8
D - 66121 Saarbrücken
Telefax: +49 681 93 81 567-9

info@omniscriptum.com
www.omniscriptum.com

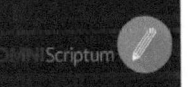

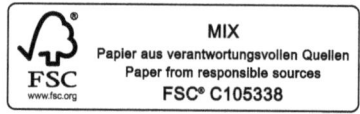

Printed by Books on Demand GmbH, Norderstedt / Germany